To Kaki
With Many Blessings!
Janet Greer

The Nana Stories

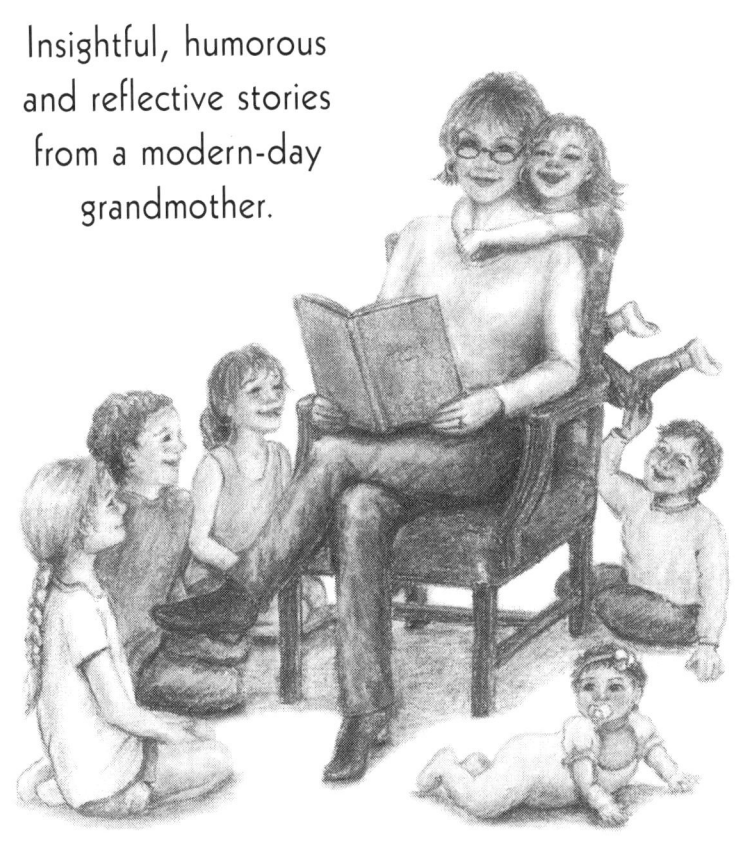

Insightful, humorous
and reflective stories
from a modern-day
grandmother.

Janet Greer

Copyright © Janet L. Greer. All rights reserved.
Manuscript Copyright © 2014 by Janet L. Greer
Cover Illustration © 2014 Lisa Haggerty Palmer
Layout: Elizabeth Fisher

No part of this book may be reproduced, stored in a retrieval system, or transmitted by any means without the written permission of the author.

Janet L. Greer
www.janetlgreer.com
Contact: janet@janetlgreer.com

First Printing, October 2014

ISBN: 978-0-9910060-1-4 (sc)
ISBN: 978-0-9910060-2-1 (e)

Printed in the United States of America

Dedication

To the most wonderful daughters a mother could ask for and the amazing young men they chose to be a part of our family. Thank you Kristy and Brant and Jenny and Bradley for giving your Pop and me six of the greatest blessings in our life.

Allie
Sawyer
Chase
Greer
Cohen
Piper

Contents

Introduction

Our Family Tree

Chapter One .... What's In a Name?

Chapter Two .... It Never Gets Old
　　　　　　　　　　　— The Birth of a Grandchild

Chapter Three .... Grandchildren Do and Say the
　　　　　　　　　　　Darnedest Things

Chapter Four .... Potty Humor

Chapter Five .... Holiday Hoopla

Chapter Six .... Sometimes It Just Hurts

Chapter Seven .... The Gift of Time
　　　　　　　　　　　and Making Memories

Acknowledgements

Our Family Tree

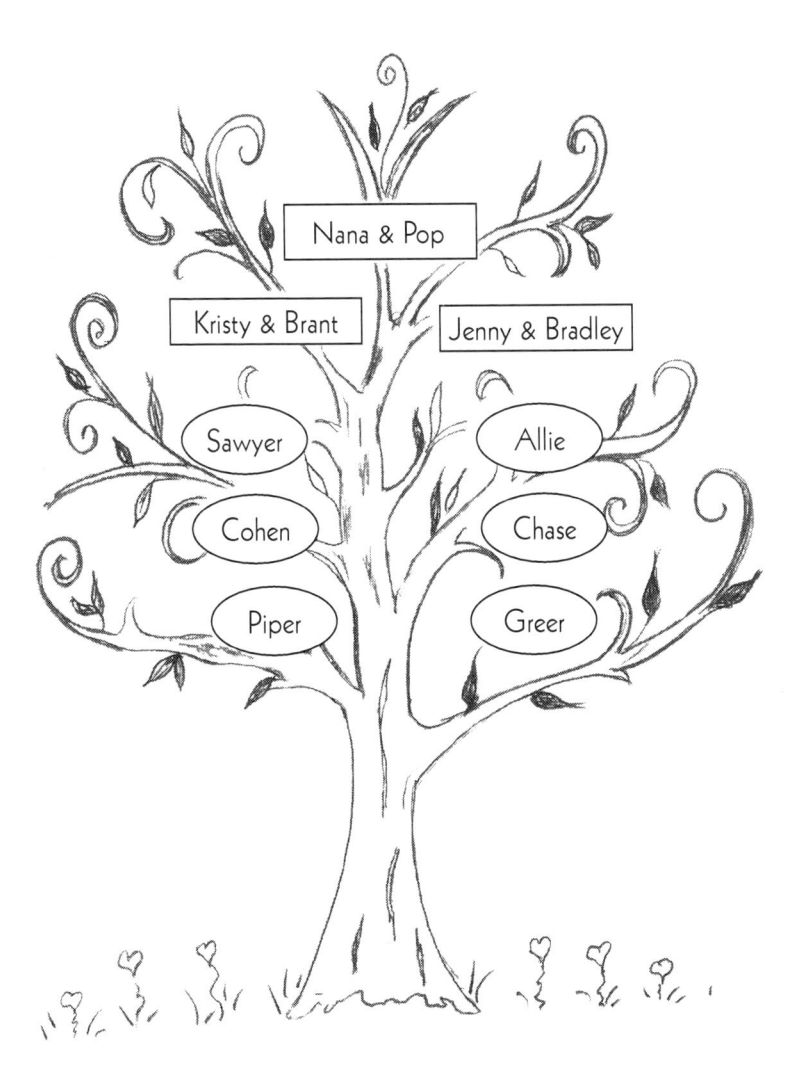

- Nana & Pop
  - Kristy & Brant
    - Sawyer
    - Cohen
    - Piper
  - Jenny & Bradley
    - Allie
    - Chase
    - Greer

Introduction

I have waited almost my entire adult life to become a grandmother. The thought of having little bundles of joy to love and spoil just made me giddy with excitement. I truly couldn't wait.

However, it would be quite a few years before finally receiving the announcement that every grandparent-to-be longs for. I was going to be a grandmother!

The news was made even sweeter when my husband and I learned both of our daughters, Kristy and Jenny, were going to have babies within three months of each other.

I was one happy gal.

As it turns out, within a span of five years our family grew to include five precious grandchildren. Recently, we added one more, and I call the six of them The Grands.

And, they call me Nana.

As you can imagine, with six grandchildren there is always something going on that is news worthy, at least in our little world. Almost every day, sometimes more than once, I am sharing a story about something that one of my six have done or said.

My husband Russell, known as Pop to our daughters and The Grands, gets a daily report. I also have a friend who calls me once a week. She wants the latest on what the most mischievous one of our six grandchildren has done to send her mama—and Nana—into a tail spin.

I am never ever at a loss for words when it comes to talking about The Grands. I love my husband and daughters beyond reason, but those precious little darlings add an extra twinkle to my eyes.

If you are a grandparent like me, you know exactly what I am talking about. You also know that we can laugh out loud at our grandchildren's antics or snicker behind our hand at some of the outrageous things they do because, after all, at the end of the day, we get to send them home.

In spite of the occasional chaos that envelopes our home when all of The Grands visit, I must say that I wouldn't trade one moment of it for anything. The time I spend with my grandchildren is priceless.

I do need to explain to you that this book is not fiction. Every bit of what I have to tell you is true. I have not made any of this stuff up. And, by the way, I do have permission to share these stories with you. This was a must because I want to continue unsupervised visits with my grandchildren in the future.

So thank you for allowing me the privilege of sharing with you some of my Nana stories. They are mostly humorous, often thoughtful and sometimes reflective. At the end of the day I hope to bring you laughter, encouragement and the assurance that we, as grandparents, have been given a golden opportunity to make a difference in the life of some very special beings. Let's make every moment count.

Now grab your favorite beverage, sit back, and enjoy The Nana Stories, as I introduce my family to yours. JG

Grandchildren are God's way of compensating us for growing old.

—May Waldrip

Chapter One
What's in a Name?

Grandmothers have certainly changed over the years. Modern day versions barely resemble the ones I grew up with. And the titles, oh my goodness! Some of my friends put more thought into what they want their grandchildren to call them than they do their Last Will and Testament.

We'll chat more about that later.

It is impossible to write about my experiences as a Nana without reflecting back on my own grandmothers. My memories of them are wonderful. I was very young when my Mamaw passed away so I don't have as many memories about her. What I do recall was that she had a whole bunch of kids. Eleven to be exact.

Mamaw, like most women in those days, worked really hard caring for her large family. She and Papaw grew most all of their food and that meant canning and preserving, which is incredibly hard work if you have never done it. The other thing I remember was her washing machine.

On washing day, Mamaw's routine was to roll a wringer washer from the back porch into the kitchen and use a hose to get water from the faucet to the tub of the washer. After the wash cycle she would ring each piece of clothing one at a time through this wringer (the equivalent of two rolling pins rotating counter clockwise) to get the soap out. Next she would drain the water out and replace it with clean water. She then put the soapy clothes back into the rinse water, one piece at a time, before running the clothes back through the wringer to get the water out.

Mamaw wasn't done yet.

After all that, she would haul a metal tub full of wet clothes up a hill to the clothes line. One by one, she hung each piece on the line with wooden clothes pins. If it was a sunny day it took only half a day to dry a load of clothes.

When the clothes were dry, she would put them all back in the metal tub and cart them back down the hill. Here is the most awful part. She had to iron most of the clothes. And, although Mamaw had electricity, she used a flat iron that was heated on top of the stove.

I am so grateful for modern appliances!

My other grandmother was called Granny, and she was my favorite. This was mostly because she liked to wear red lipstick and dress up. I remember her wearing a two-piece suit and pill box hat every time she went downtown to shop at Miller's Department Store. I don't think I ever saw a gray hair on her head and she lived into her nineties. Thank goodness for hair color in a box.

Granny was only about five feet tall at best, and she

wore black cat-eye shaped glasses. She always wore an apron around the house, too. Funny thing was, as concerned about her appearance as she was, she still kept a toothpick in her mouth most of the time. This toothpick was not one of those little skinny things you pick up in restaurants. It was a hickory stick about three inches long that she would cut from a tree in her yard.

Granny would use this homemade toothpick to dip snuff out of a tiny little snuff box and place it in her mouth. My mama told me that Granny used to smoke cigarettes in her younger days but later, when smoking became unacceptable for women in public places, she switched to dipping snuff.

I'm a lot like my Granny. I have her short stature, I love to dress up, and I also wear bright lipstick. While I don't use the same brand of hair color, I do admit to covering my gray. However, I promise I have never had the desire to put a toothpick with snuff on it in my mouth nor will I ever. I prefer chocolate instead.

~ ❤ ~

I now return to the subject of how one decides what to be called by their grandchildren. Many of my friends decided to be called the same name as their favorite grandmother, mostly because they have warm and fuzzy memories associated with that person.

When I found out I was to be a grandmother for the first time, I began to contemplate what I wanted to be called. My husband Russell was already called Pop by our daughters so I decided my grandparent label needed to complement his.

However, the more I thought about it, the more I struggled. I did not want to be called Granny or Mamaw even if that was what my two grandmothers were called.

They were old and I am not!

So what was a not-so-old, modern, hip and fun grandmother to be called? After all, I wear skirts above the knee, blue jeans on occasion, a fair amount of make-up and dangly earrings. Oh yeah, I like bright polish on my toenails too. These are things my two grandmothers would have never done, except the red lipstick, of course.

After way too much thought, I decided I wanted to be called Nana. One would assume that it was because Nana and Pop sound so cute together and they do. Yet I have to confess it was because if one of The Grands shouted out "Nana!" in public, I figured it would sound like Anna.

Truthfully, that was my thinking at the time.

But let me tell you this. The first time I laid eyes on my precious granddaughter and introduced myself to her as Nana, my heart grew a thousand times. She could have called me Miss Dirt Bag after that, and I would have thought it the greatest name in the world.

It quickly became evident that I didn't care what she called me as long as she called me. Period.

As I have learned, some grandmothers don't have a choice in what they are called by their grandchildren, despite good intentions. When a young child starts jabbering and learning to talk, they don't always hear what you are saying or they translate words in a different way. Once they start calling you by the name of their choosing, there is no going back.

THE NANA STORIES

Whatever the heck the little dumplings decide to call you, from that point on, you are stuck with it. Nonetheless, if you are a grandmother-to-be reading this and need some suggestions for a nickname, here are just a few that friends and family were kind enough to share with me.

Granny	Gram	Gramma	Grammy
Grandma	Grandy	Ga Ga	Gamma
Ginnie	Gran Gran	Granny	Gigi
G-Ma	Grandmama	Granna	GrAnn
Gabby	Happy	Mimi	Mamaw
Memaw	Maw	Nanny	Nana
Nenaw	Dee Dee	Chickie	Baba
Nana Banana	Nona (Italian)	Ruby Shoes	Nina
Farmore (Swedish)	Nay Nay		

One of my favorite submissions was Lolly. The grandmother who shared it with me said it stands for "Little Old Lady Loves You." I love that.

I also received the following suggestions for grandfathers:

Pop	Poppy	Papa	Poppee
Granddad	Granddaddy	Papaw	Pappy
Mustache	Big Daddy	Daddy Mike	Paw
Pigi	P-Paw	Partner	Papaw
Grandpop	Grandpa		

What's in a name? It really doesn't matter. You will love your new name no matter how silly it may sound or how little sense it makes to you. What matters most is that we, the grandparent, can take the very best of who we are to help make it a part of who our grandchildren become. That is our legacy.

Grandparents are a delightful blend of laughter, caring deeds, wonderful stories and love.

—Author Unknown

Chapter Two
It Never Gets Old – The Birth of a Grandchild

I never thought I would be blessed with another grandchild before I completed the manuscript for The Nana Stories, but that's what happened. My two daughters, Kristy and Jenny, had informed me their families were complete. I believed them.

Our family included five absolutely precious grandchildren, but there I was, on my way to Georgia to be with my first born who was about to deliver her third child, a girl.

Kristy has two boys and really wanted another son, but God had a different plan. Keep in mind Kristy does not like change. She knew what to do with boys after all. According to her, boys are easy. Girls would be more work.

"Besides," she once told me, "I don't like the color pink." After finding out this new addition was to be a girl, she even put on her gift registry "No Pink."

No kidding.

I don't mind telling you I was concerned about this. I had my motherly speech ready to reassure Kristy that having a girl was going to be okay. I had two of my own so I should know what I was talking about. In my mature and infinite wisdom I suspected her concern wasn't so much that she was having a girl but that she was adding another little one to their family.

Where would she find the energy to take care of a third child and still hold down a full-time job? Would there be room enough in her heart for another?

I am happy to say that as soon as that sweet perfect baby girl was born, her mother fell in love all over again. Piper was beautiful and healthy, and it turns out there was plenty of room in Kristy's heart for one more.

It was a wonderful sight to behold. The precious little bundle even came home in the same outfit her mama had worn as she too left the hospital more than 36 years ago.

And, it had tiny *pink* roses on it.

This story gets even better. After arriving home, Kristy asked me to change Piper's clothes. Well, it just so happened that I found a pretty little pink outfit hidden in the dresser drawer. There was even a pink cap with a bow on top.

I didn't say a word as I returned the sleeping child, all in pink, to her bassinet. Her mother took one look at her daughter and said, "Huh. She looks really good in pink."

Go figure.

~♥~

At the birth of each of my grandchildren, I couldn't help but think back to the ones who had been born before. The first granddaughter was the most anticipated because, well, she was the first. I remember it well because the call came in that my daughter Jenny was in labor while I was at a candlelight service at the cemetery where my parents were laid to rest.

This was a bittersweet moment because I knew I wouldn't get to share the birth of my first grandchild with them.

At any rate, as is usual, births are rarely convenient. Bradley, our son-in-law, had also called his parents. The other grandparents-to-be, B.J. and Mike, happened to be hosting a holiday party at their home that evening. They had a house full of guests when they received the call to come to the hospital. Ever the perfect hosts, and not wanting to spoil the party for their guests, they merely asked that someone lock up when the party ended.

The in-laws headed to the hospital where they joined Pop and me as we waited for our first grandchild to be born. Allie came to us in the early morning hours one week before Christmas. Oh, what a gift! She was here, she was healthy, and she was beautiful.

All of us were off on a magical journey of love, cuddles, laughter and more. This first little Grand taught me how to be a grandparent and paved the way for the rest of them. I only had to open my heart and let all the wonderful moments pour in.

~♥~

Three months later our second grandchild, Sawyer, arrived almost too soon. Kristy was scheduled to be induced two weeks early because of pregnancy and baby complications. She and her husband, Brant, lived two states away, so I drove down the day before to be with them for the blessed event.

I awoke that next morning with my daughter telling me we

didn't have to leave for the hospital for another couple hours.

However, one look at Kristy and I knew something was not quite right. This being her first child, Kristy didn't know any better, but I did. She was already in labor, and I mean hard labor.

I suggested she get dressed—she was still in her pajamas—and that we should head to the hospital right away. She argued that we couldn't go for two more hours until they had room for her. Instinct told me we didn't have two hours. If Kristy followed my pattern of childbirth, she would have the baby sooner rather than later. As it turned out I was right.

The car ride to the hospital was not a long one but it seemed to take forever. Fortunately, it was early morning and there wasn't much traffic. I really believed we might be delivering the baby in the car.

Brant let us out at the door and as soon as we walked in I explained to the receptionist that my daughter was about to have her baby. This was a women's hospital where patients took an elevator directly up to the labor and delivery floor. Kristy was offered a wheelchair but she refused. She couldn't sit.

As we exited the elevator the nurse's station was only about twenty feet away, but Kristy was having to stop every few feet because of the pain. I called out that we needed help, explaining that my daughter was in hard labor and that this baby was at risk for complications.

If only you could have seen the look on the faces of the staff. I could just hear them saying, oh good gracious, we've got a hysterical mama on our hands.

The nurse explained they did not have any birthing rooms

available and they would just have to put Kristy on one of the extra beds at the end of the hall. By this time, Brant had arrived from parking the car so we all crowded into this make-shift delivery room, literally in a hallway. A staff member had the courtesy, at least, to pull a portable screen in front of Kristy's bed to allow some privacy.

A few minutes later a nurse assistant explained to us that she needed to examine Kristy to see how far she had dilated. The lady proceeded to take her sweet time, moving as slow as molasses.

What happened next was like something out of a movie. If the situation hadn't been so serious it would have looked like a comedy being played out. I can laugh about it now but, in truth, it still sends shivers up my spine knowing all the things that could have gone wrong.

The assistant proceeded to check Kristy and then, all of a sudden, she shouted, "Oh, honey, you're at ten!" She turned and literally ran back down the hall.

Then I heard my scared daughter start to cry.

Being first time parents-to-be, Kristy and Brant had taken childbirth classes so they would be prepared for the birth of their child. They wanted everything to be textbook perfect. Kristy was a teacher after all, and that was how it is supposed to be. However, because she had taken the class, she knew ten centimeters meant no drugs. They had planned for an epidural.

By this time the nurse assistant had informed everyone at the nurse's station about the results of Kristy's pelvic exam. That's when, excuse the expression, all hell broke loose.

People with carts came flying down the hall from all

directions. Gowns were being put on, instruments unwrapped, and an incubator for the baby was placed nearby. I was just outside the screen, flattened up against the wall, trying to stay out of the way.

While all the personnel available were working within the confines of that small space, preparing for the birth of my grandson, another gentleman came sauntering down the hall. One look at the name on his lab coat confirmed he was the anesthesiologist. He looked at me and asked, "Who are you?" I replied, "I'm the Mama." He then poked his head into the controlled chaos surrounding my daughter and asked how things were going.

The nurse said, "Oh, she's at ten and completely effaced."

I will never forget this. The doctor calmly replied, "Well, you don't need me." He turned away and walked right back down the hall.

At this news, Kristy let out a loud cry which was my cue to leave. I was not about to stand in that hall and listen as my daughter experienced natural childbirth.

Except for the trauma of a very fast delivery— in a hallway no less—I can tell you that everything turned out fine. I became the proud Nana of a healthy baby boy named Sawyer, and Kristy wasn't so traumatized that she refused to have any more children. In fact, two more came along later.

And yes, an epidural was involved.

Things don't always go the way they are supposed to, just like Sawyer's quick arrival almost without warning. It seems our family has had our share of unexpected incidents involving the birth of our grandchildren.

When my other daughter Jenny had her second baby, she too followed the path of rapid deliveries. A blessing to be sure but sometimes childbirth happens a little too fast for the good of the babe. This was the case with Chase.

All seemed to be going well after her arrival. Chase was being cuddled by her great uncle when suddenly the little booger's face turned a scary shade of purple. Not normal.

Her daddy, Bradley, ran down the hall to get a nurse who proceeded to turn Chase upside down and pound on, okay, firmly pat on her back, until she coughed up a large amount of mucus. Apparently, when a baby travels down the birth canal too fast, Mother Nature is prevented from squeezing all of the gunk out of the little one's lungs.

After a night in the nursery being monitored, our third grandchild was declared perfect, much to the relief of us all.

Later when I recounted this story to a now six-year-old Chase, she replied with a broad smile, "Maybe that's why I'm a fast runner!"

We've decided this one will be a future track star.

~♥~

Our fourth grandchild, Greer, recently turned four. In her honor we held a small family dinner that included all her favorite foods. Dessert was chocolate layer cake with hazelnut frosting, whipped cream and strawberries. She pranced around with her new tiara perched on her little blonde head, waving her matching fairy wand and wearing a set of beautiful fairy wings that twinkled.

She was in her element.

Watching her pixie little self brought so much delight, especially when I recall her entry into this world. A couple years after Chase was born we were thrilled to be told another Grand was on the way. Jenny and Bradley were pretty happy too. It was the first of their three children that was actually planned. Birth control pills and antibiotics don't mix.

Everything was going to be by the book this time. Her pregnancy progressed well until sixteen weeks. By that time, it was determined this baby had IUGR (intrauterine growth restriction). In layman's terms, her tiny body wasn't growing as it should.

By the last trimester of Jenny's pregnancy, it was determined that this baby's chances of survival were best outside the womb. The decision was made to induce her as soon as possible. Jenny was at thirty-four weeks of gestation at this point. The induction was scheduled the very next day.

The timing couldn't have come at a worse time for me personally. I had just had an abnormal mammogram that same day, and I was to return at the end of the week for additional tests. I did not share this with Jenny. I didn't want any shadow cast on the birth of this baby, especially not knowing if she was going to be born with complications.

The day of baby Greer's birth came. There were no complications in the delivery, and she came into this world weighing four pounds, six ounces. She was labeled a preemie but she appeared normal and was doing well. Everything checked out okay at this point, so we celebrated.

With much excitement, Greer's two big sisters came to visit. They were decked out in personalized shirts that said I'm Greer's Biggest Sister and I'm Greer's Big Sister. The nurses put hair nets and gloves on the two girls, and they were adorable. Allie and Chase both agreed that their baby sister was a keeper.

However, our euphoria didn't last.

Later that day Greer began to experience respiratory problems. Her lungs were not fully developed and she couldn't regulate her body temperature. The decision was made to transport her to the neonatal intensive care unit at the local children's hospital. There she could receive the best care possible. This was upsetting to us, but heart wrenching for my daughter and son-in-law.

Jenny and Bradley had to watch as a team of personnel from the unit came and took away their tiny baby girl. It was a pitiful site. The portable incubator looked like an extra-large see-through box with oxygen feeding into it. Inside was our itty-bitty Greer. That picture is one that continues to haunt me.

The next morning my husband Russell accompanied me to my appointment at the breast center. I thought I had a strong faith, but I have to tell you I was more than a little scared about what the results of another mammogram and ultrasound would determine.

As it turned out the breast center was just a block away from the children's hospital where our preemie granddaughter had been taken. When I was finished at the breast center, we immediately went to the hospital to see Greer.

En route, Russell made the decision not to go onto

the unit. He didn't think he could handle seeing his newest granddaughter in that environment. I certainly wasn't prepared for what awaited me.

After scrubbing in for what seemed like forever I was escorted into the neonatal intensive care unit, past lots of tiny beds with very sick infants. Soon I stood in front of our sweet baby Greer and saw that she was hooked up to all kinds of monitors. There were tubes in her nose and her mouth, and needles in places I don't even want to describe.

My heart just about broke. All it took for the dam to break was seeing Jenny, sitting by her little girl's tiny bed, holding onto an itty-bitty finger.

Of course, one look at me and Jenny lost it. That was when I knew it was time to put my big girl panties on and be the mama this girl needed right now. Bradley seemed to be holding up, but it has been my experience that men do not do well in situations like this. They have no control over any of it, and they can't fix it.

I was only allowed a very short visit with Greer, and the time quickly passed. It was hard leaving the baby and her parents, but my mind was occupied with the results of my pending test. I now have three granddaughters along with my two daughters, two sisters and a bunch of nieces.

I continued my silent prayer. *Please Lord don't let me have breast cancer.*

Later that day I received the news that all of my tests were clean. Hallelujah!

Those were some scary days. Greer's spunky spirit served her well and she was so very lucky to have only minimal long-term effects from being born premature. Although she is still a tiny thing for her age, she brings much laughter with her constant antics, as well as anxiety at times because of her mischievous behavior and her fearless take-no-prisoners attitude.

All the things that Greer does to drive her parents crazy now will serve her well into adulthood, I'm quite sure. That being said, we love her to pieces and can't imagine life without her.

~♥~

After the traumatic birth of her first son, I wasn't sure my daughter Kristy would ever want to have another child. However, one day while I was checking my email, I noticed a message from her. The subject line was "A Picture from Sawyer." My grandson, who was about four and a half years old at the time, wasn't much into art so I was intrigued.

When I opened the attachment it wasn't art. It was a photograph of him holding a flash card that read, "We're having a baby!" Needless to say I was shocked by the news, but also very excited.

Fortunately, this pregnancy was quite normal. Cohen, our fifth grandchild, arrived into this world a very healthy little boy. His mother had a little bit of drama afterwards with some postpartum complications, but within a few days all was good.

Our family welcomed this adorable boy with big blue eyes and dimpled cheeks into our hearts. It is the memory of his sweetness in those early days that allow us to love him unconditionally now.

While Cohen is still cute as a button, he is very strong

willed and never still. This tiny tornado keeps us on our toes and his parents on their knees.

~♥~

I started this chapter with the birth of our sixth grandchild, Piper. She has dark hair, a dimpled chin and blue gray eyes. She too made a hasty entrance into this world.

Kristy was having some blood pressure issues late in the pregnancy so things were being monitored closely. After several hours of observation in the hospital on a Friday afternoon, it was decided that she would be on bed rest at home for the weekend and would be re-evaluated at the first of the week.

At the doctor's office that Monday morning, it was determined her blood pressure had not stabilized with bed rest, so an induction was necessary. I headed down to Georgia even though Kristy assured me I didn't have to hurry. However, given her past history, I wasn't buying it.

On arriving at the hospital and walking into Kristy's room, I took one look at her and knew something was not right. I was thinking, here we go again.

Kristy looked at me and said, "I can't feel my arms."

A quick look at the monitor where her vitals were being recorded showed that her blood pressure was nowhere near normal and her heart rate was too high.

I called for the nurse and several members of the staff began to work with her. In addition, Kristy's labor was picking up. Her doctor was called, and it was determined they would stop the drug that induces labor because it was contributing to her blood pressure issues and her labor was progressing quickly enough on her own.

That was putting it mildly.

Kristy began to feel a lot of pressure. In addition, her epidural had stopped working at this point. Her doctor was notified but was having to commute from another area hospital. Minutes ticked by and things quickly progressed. The nurses kept calling the doctor and began to gather the medical supplies necessary to deliver in the room.

At this point, I was expecting a nurse would deliver the baby since there still was no doctor, and I knew Kristy could not wait much longer. I couldn't help but be reminded of her firstborn being delivered in a hallway. At least, this time she was in a room.

Suddenly, I hear the sound of someone running down the hall. Kristy's doctor comes barreling in, removing her jacket and holding out her arms for a nurse to shove some gloves on her. That was my exit cue.

Earlier in the day I had called Russell to let him know what was happening. He was nearing the hospital and phoned for directions as to where to meet me. I instructed him to come to the waiting area where we would wait together for news. He and I arrived at the waiting area at about the same time and sat down.

While I was bringing Russell up-to-date on everything that had happened with Kristy, I received a text message. I looked down and there was the face of our brand new granddaughter just a few minutes old.

With tears in my eyes and my heart bursting with joy, I shared the photo with Russell. Quietly I said, "Oh my, it never gets old."

You now have an introduction to my six amazing grandchildren. Allie, Sawyer, Chase, Greer, Cohen and Piper. In the coming pages you will learn so much as you enjoy the antics and revelations of their very different personalities.

I wouldn't change anything about The Grands, even though a couple of them would challenge a saint. However, there is no doubt in my mind that each will grow up to be incredibly caring, creative and loving individuals.

> *Perfect love sometimes does not come until the first grandchild.*
>
> —Welsh Proverb

Chapter Three
Grandchildren Do and Say the Darnedest Things

Anyone Have a Loose Tooth?

My first grandson Sawyer is a pretty smart kid. At four years of age he was downloading games from his parents' smart phone. They didn't realize it until they received the charges on their monthly cell phone statement.

Their phones are now password protected.

Sawyer also helps me when I can't figure out how to use my phone or computer. It's amazing. Another thing he does is record all kinds of kid-friendly programs on our DVR when visiting our home. He also deletes some of our pre-recorded programs. I guess he needed the room.

With Sawyer's knack for electronics, I was thinking this was a good thing. Maybe his future is in the internet technology industry. Techs make pretty good money and, because of technically challenged people like me, I doubt those jobs will ever become obsolete. However, with this latest turn of events, I now have my doubts that employment in the technology field is in Sawyer's future after all.

Apparently, Sawyer has the predisposition to be a thrill seeker. He keeps pulling his own loose teeth. When Sawyer figured out that other kids his age had received money under their pillow in exchange for the teeth they had lost, that was all the incentive he needed to work on that loose tooth.

It wasn't long until Sawyer had successfully pulled his first tooth. It was a proud day in my daughter's house.

Over the next couple months Sawyer lost two more teeth, again pulling them himself. How much does the Tooth Fairy pay, for goodness sakes? This kid is racking up. I am now thinking that perhaps dentistry may be his future profession.

A few days later Kristy sent me a text message to say Sawyer had pulled yet another tooth, this one on the top. Then, I kid you not, about two hours later on the very same day I received a picture on my phone. Sawyer had pulled tooth number five. He looked like a jack-o'-lantern.

Again, I ask, what does that Tooth Fairy pay?

I'm Sorry

Our second grandson Cohen started out as a sweet, roly-poly little fellow with big blue eyes, dimples and a smile that will get him just about anything he wants. He stole our hearts from the get-go. However, Cohen, now three years old, is becoming somewhat of a challenge. He is big for his age and very strong-willed.

Truth be known, I think he has been taking private lessons in bad behavior from Greer. However, Cohen still charms the pants off us but we are getting a little bit wiser.

While Cohen is a little aggressive, his big brother is not. Sawyer is a sweet, caring young man who has been taught not to hit or be mean to his baby brother.

Big mistake. One such instance was when Cohen decided to whack his brother for no apparent reason. He hit Sawyer in the face and made him cry. Kristy, Cohen's mother, witnessed the act, picked him up and explained it was not nice to hit. He would have to go to time-out. This meant Cohen would have to sit in a chair away from everyone for a couple of minutes.

By the way, I sure wish my parents had known about time-out when I was little.

At any rate, when the minutes had passed, Kristy reiterated to Cohen again, "We do not hit," and she instructed him to say he was sorry.

Obviously, she meant for Cohen to tell Sawyer he was sorry for hitting him. Cohen looked his mother straight in the eye and stated emphatically, "I'm sorry you're Cohen's mommy!"

I was nearby and it was all I could do to keep a straight face, especially after seeing the stunned look on Kristy's face. Priceless.

It's All Greer

At the risk of slighting my other grandchildren, these next few stories are about Greer. It's not that I'm partial to her, it's just that there is hardly a day that goes by that she doesn't say or do something noteworthy. The girl never stops. Ever.

I have also learned one very important thing to remember

about Greer. Never take your eyes off of her. As my story continues, you will soon understand this comment. This girl is becoming infamous, and she's not even five years old.

Look Nana, I Painted!

Like all grandparents, I believe my grandchildren to be the smartest, most beautiful, talented and exceptional beings God ever created. While they each have their own gifts and personalities, it gives me great pleasure that Allie, Chase and Greer seem to have inherited my creative flare. Because of this, no matter their ages, I have attempted to introduce them to different craft projects when they are in my care.

As this story progresses, keep in mind their ages at the time. Allie is seven, Chase is five-and-a-half, and Greer is two-and-a-half.

Some days, when visiting Nana's house, the girls and I bake cookies. They can't be just plain cookies; they have to have icing and sprinkles. The bigger mess we make, the better the cookies.

The other favorite thing my granddaughters like to do is play dress-up. They have more princess dresses, boas, jewels (pretend ones, of course) and fancy slippers than you can imagine.

On top of that, each one of them loves to perform. With microphones made of hair brushes and ice cream scoops, dressed to the nines, they sing and dance for us.

It's cheap entertainment.

However, on very special days with Nana, they are allowed to enter my studio to paint with me. It is a hobby that brings me much pleasure. I also love sharing this passion with my grandchildren. Allie, Chase and Greer enjoy painting also. They understand it is a great day at Nana's house when they get to paint.

There is just one condition. They are never to go into the studio without me.

Each of them, or so I thought, understood this to the point that I have not needed to put a lock on the studio door. For the most part, The Grands are well-behaved children, but remember what I said about Greer. Never take your eyes off of her.

It wasn't anything new that my granddaughters loved crafting and painting with me. However, I was surprised when my oldest grandson Sawyer showed some interest. He is more into boy toys and video games. So imagine my delight when shopping at the local craft store, I found a small canvas that had a pre-printed pirate ship on it. Sawyer just happened to be into pirates at the time.

Perfect.

The next time he visited, Sawyer and I set up in the studio for some quality painting time together. He really seemed to enjoy the special time with Nana. Unfortunately, he was unable to finish painting his small canvas before he left to go home. I promised that when he returned for his next visit we would finish it since he was excited he would have something he painted hanging in his room. I left the unfinished canvas, clean brushes and tubes of paint on the table and closed the door.

About a week later my daughter Jenny, along with Allie, Chase and Greer, came for lunch. While Jenny and I chatted at the kitchen table, the girls asked permission to go to the playroom upstairs. This is allowed without supervision because, as I said before, they are well-behaved children.

However, the last thing I said was, "Allie and Chase, let us know if Greer gets into anything you know she shouldn't be doing." I apparently chose to ignore what I mentioned earlier about Greer. Never take your eyes off her.

Jenny and I were deep in conversation and enjoying the summer sunshine streaming into the kitchen. All of a sudden we hear this sweet, yet excited, voice proclaiming, "Nana, I painted!"

With a look of terror on my face I bolted up the stairs, ran down the hall to my open studio door, and froze. There sat Greer with a look of pure delight on her face and a paint brush in her hand.

In my heart I was overjoyed at the scene in front of me, and I didn't dare scold her. But, in my head, I am thinking, oh my gosh! However, all that came out of my mouth was, "Greer, don't move!"

The next thing was a shout. "Jenny come help me!"

Greer had decided to take advantage of the lack of supervision—a mistake on our part—to express her artistic self. She painted all over the unfinished canvas left by Sawyer. She must like pirate ships too.

Greer continued her new-found creativity on both her hands, both arms, her face and her pretty little white eyelet top. And, did I mention the only tube of paint she managed to open was black?

As I was trying to get her top off without getting any

THE NANA STORIES

more paint on it, I realized the situation had become worse.

At this point in time, Greer was not quite potty trained. I suppose, in her need for intense concentration on her art project, she forgot she needed to go to the bathroom. Greer stunk to high heaven. By this time Jenny had come into the room, took a whiff, and said, "Forget the clothes, we have to get this pull-up off of her!"

Fortunately, there was an adjoining bath next to the studio. Greer happily laid on the floor while her mama continued to get her clean.

Greer looked up and made eye contact with me. I still can see the expression on her face that said, "Look, Nana I painted!" She was so proud. But, even a Nana has to scold sometimes. I was very stern as I reminded Greer that she was not to ever go in the studio without me again. Secretly, I was pleased at her efforts.

I put a lock on the door after that.

Now, all that was left to do was get rid of Greer's masterpiece. I must not leave any evidence.

Because my grandson had never before expressed any desire to paint, I was hopeful he would never ask about the pirate canvas. That wasn't to be. I thought that disaster had been put to rest until, six months later, Sawyer came to visit. I kid you not, he asked me if he could finish his pirate ship painting.

Uh oh. I have some explaining to do.

Still, to this day, I can't walk into that room without seeing tiny little Greer, sitting on her knees in the chair with brush in hand. Who knows, maybe one day when she is grown she will paint a true masterpiece, call me up and say, "Look Nana, I painted!"

Talk like a Duck

One day a week I pick Greer up from preschool. It is interesting spending time with her without Allie and Chase. Greer is definitely her own person and is never lacking for something to talk about. This particular day as we were driving back to her house, she seemed unusually quiet. This was not like her at all.

Greer may have just been tired, so I decided to perk her up a bit. There is one thing I do with all The Grands that always brings a laugh. I talk like a duck. So I pretended to sneeze, and it came out in my duck voice.

Well, instead of laughing as usual, Greer just made eye contact with me in the rear view mirror and said, "Can you do that in Spanish?"

And no, I haven't figured out how to talk like a duck in Spanish. I must be getting old.

I Just Want to Look Fabulous

Once again, on a trip home from preschool, Greer wanted to share with me how her day at school went. She began the conversation in a very matter-of-fact manner.

"Mary doesn't pinch her mommy. She only pinches little kids."

I replied, "Oh my. Did she pinch you?"

"Yes, when I was in time-out," Greer said.

Trying not to smile, I asked, "Why were you in time-out?"

Greer continued to explain, "I hit Tommy."

"Why did you hit Tommy?"

"He hit me first."

"Did you tell the teacher?"

After a short pause she answered, "No." Her response told me there might be more to this story than she had said.

I decided to change the subject. Earlier when I was helping her get into the car, I noticed that sometime during the day, Greer had apparently decided to use markers to draw lines up and down both of her forearms. I asked her why she thought it was a good idea to do this.

She replied, "I just want to look fabulous."

Daring to go a bit further with this conversation I asked, "What are the large colored dots on both of your palms?"

Greer answered, "Oh, those are for my fire power."

I didn't even want to know why she thought she needed fire power.

Death by Fairy Wand

Earlier, in a previous chapter, I mentioned that Greer loves dressing up. She will put on some of the most outrageous outfits you have ever seen. The only thing Greer likes as much as dressing up is dancing around the room.

One afternoon, decked out in a favorite tutu and brandishing a fairy wand with streamers, she proceeded to prance and dance all over the place.

Greer's interpretive movements are extraordinary to say the least. Arms and legs go every which way. It is something to behold.

On this particular day, she was whirling and twirling in the family room where her daddy's pride and joy was located. This would be a sixty-inch plasma television that he had purchased during his bachelor days. It was one impressive piece of entertainment with a price tag to match.

Caught up in the moment of her performance, Greer swung her arms around and accidentally hit the television with her fairy wand.

Now this was Greer's version of what happened. Her mama has another. Jenny states the attack was totally deliberate and unprovoked. Either way, the television met its demise that fateful day.

The assault by the fairy wand-welding Greer did not break the glass surface of the television. However, it did make the screen have only a partial picture and squiggly lines. The TV doctor had to be consulted, and the diagnosis was not good. The damage was terminal and the beloved television had to be put down.

Jenny swears she could hear sobbing coming from the other end of the phone when she called Bradley to break the sad news. The cause of death was determined to be death by fairy wand.

A Bad Idea

A few years ago our entire family went to an amusement park. It was great fun. Pop and I loved seeing the faces of The Grands each time they spotted one of their favorite characters. It is truly a magical place, with the exception of one ride.

My son-in-law Brant was the biggest "kid" there. He

didn't want to miss a thing, and both he and Sawyer experienced more than any of the rest of us.

Before the trip even began they talked about a particular ride in the park. Sawyer's cousin, a girl, had ridden it earlier in the year and pronounced it great fun. Well, if a girl could ride it and live to tell about it, so could he.

Sawyer's dad was behind the idea one hundred percent. His mom not so much. Kristy thought Sawyer was too young. However, when they approached the entrance to the ride, they found Sawyer actually met the height requirement.

To my surprise, Pop decided to go along as well. He is not much into amusement rides, but I think his presence was for backup in the event Sawyer decided to back out at the last minute. Or, more importantly, it might make Sawyer feel more comfortable about getting on the ride.

The entire time the boys were off on their adventure, Kristy and I waited nearby. She was very uncomfortable about Sawyer riding the ride. She warned Brant that if their son was traumatized by the ride, he—Brant—was going to be in big trouble.

The wait seemed forever but finally, we saw the boys making their way back through the crowd to where we were waiting. Sawyer, wide-eyed, came straight over to Kristy and me. I asked him how he liked the ride.

He very mechanically replied, "It was the best ride ever." After a brief pause, Sawyer continued, "And my dad told me to tell you that."

Uh, oh.

Kristy's eyes blazed at Brant with an I-told-you-so look, but he just stood there like a deer caught in the head lights.

Pop finally broke the ice by bursting out laughing. I don't think anyone else thought it was funny.

He went on to tell us the rest of the story.

Apparently, the ride takes you up to a dizzying height in a simulated elevator. The elevator then free falls to the ground, not once, but several times. Pop explained that Sawyer never opened his mouth, to scream or otherwise. He just stood frozen between his dad and his grandfather.

Pop continued with his version of what happened next.

As soon as the ride came to a stop and the elevator doors opened, Sawyer looked at his dad and said, "Dad, this was a bad idea. Get me out of here!"

Sometimes our grandchildren know better than we do.

Like Mother Like Daughter

My second daughter Jenny decided to nurse each of her three children. Observing their mother nursing their new baby sister was nothing out of the ordinary for Allie and Chase. One day, however, I received quite a surprise while visiting them when I went to find out what three-year-old Chase was doing in her room all alone.

What I saw brought me to a standstill.

Chase was sitting on her bed with her shirt pulled up, and she had one of her baby dolls at her chest. I asked her what she was doing.

She smiled real big and said, "I'm feeding my baby just like mommy." I have no doubt that Chase will probably make a terrific mother someday.

The Color Purple

From time to time I become bored with my hair. When that happens, I allow my stylist to do pretty much whatever she wants. On one particular occasion, she and I decided to change the color to a dark auburn. Afterwards I realized when out in the sun, my hair had a little bit of an eggplant tint to it.

Oh well, I thought. It will lighten up in a week or so.

A couple days after the color change, Pop and I were having lunch with our granddaughters. The waiter brought out a small bowl of purple grapes for the girls to share.

Allie, the oldest, looked down at the grapes and proudly exclaimed, "Look Nana, these grapes are the same color as your hair!"

I made an appointment at the salon the next day.

History Repeats Itself

One day Jenny thought it was safe to take a quick shower while the three girls were watching a favorite program on television. Never a good idea. The girls decided to do something a little more entertaining. They got out markers and paper. This was usually not a problem except they decided to draw on each other instead of the paper.

Allie thought Greer would look good with a black mustache and beard. The more amazing thing is that Greer sat still long enough for Allie to do this.

Because these were washable markers, most of it came off. However, a few days afterward, you could still see the outline of a mustache on Greer. She thought it was cool because it looked like a tattoo.

The funny thing is their mama did the very same thing when she was about two years old. The difference was that markers back then were all permanent ink. Also, Jenny didn't have an accomplice. She did it all by herself. By the time I discovered her, hiding behind a door, she had drawn all over her face and up and down both arms and legs. Beautiful.

Sweet As Pie

While watching a sporting event on TV with The Grands, the crowd reacted to something that happened on the field. They weren't happy with the ruling and responded by shouting, "Booooo!"

I made the comment that booing wasn't a very nice thing to do. Allie replied, "Nana, that's not a Beatitude, that's a ME-attitude."

Well said, my sweet girl. Thank you, Sunday school teachers.

Hope It Doesn't Get Worse

When our youngest grandson Cohen started talking, he had a little trouble pronouncing some of his words. Here are a few of our favorites.

High five was "high pies." "I want a shakemilk" (milkshake). "I wanna watch a booby" (movie). The same word later became "doobie."

I sure hope we don't hear either of those words when he becomes a teen!

It's Only Logical

One day I heard Sawyer having a conversation with his mom. He apparently thought something his cousin had said was important and should be shared.

"Mom, Chase said she is a tomboy."

His mother replied, "Sawyer, do you know what a tomboy is?"

"Yes. It means she is half boy and half girl."

This and That

Allie: "Daddy cut my fingernails way too short. I can't even itch myself."

Sawyer: "The first rule is, there are no rules!"

Chase, when told she was one smart cookie: "No, I'm not. Cookies aren't smart."

Cohen, who thinks as children get bigger, adults get little like him: "Nana, when I grow up I am going to this. And, when you grow down you can do that!"

Sawyer telling his parents about a friend at school who was really smart: "He has been in the first grade twice!"

Allie: "When I grow up and be a mommy, I'm going to take my kids to preschool. Then I will go back home and have some me time."

It's funny what happens when you become a grandparent. You start to act all goofy and do things you never thought you would do. It's terrific!

—Mike Krzyzewski

Chapter Four
Potty Humor

I know this subject might not be appropriate by some folks' standards but let's face it, young children and the word "potty" always inspire funny stories. It's inevitable, especially when you have five little ones doing their thing.

Because I want The Grands to still think I'm wonderful when they are old enough to read this book, I am choosing to keep their identities anonymous in this particular section.

It's the least I can do.

Also, in order for you to completely understand some of the content of this particular chapter, I have graciously included the definition of some of the words that you will be introduced to.

Potty – going into the bathroom to do your business
Hoo Ha – girl body part
Doodle – boy body part
Booty – buttocks (also, tushy or behind)
Boobies – female breast
Pee – urine

Poo/Poop — stool
Toot — passing gas

I'm truly sorry for the visual images you now have in your head. However, this is necessary if you are to understand some of what I am about to share with you. If you are squeamish, you may want to skip this chapter. Although, if you do, you will miss a lot of laughs.

Doodle Down and Booty Call

One of my grandsons was just recently potty trained. He still uses the little portable seat that sits on top of a regular toilet seat. I had already been instructed by his mom that when I help him up on the seat, I have to hold his doodle down for him. He can't do this himself just yet. My help also prevents him from wetting his clothes.

I had been compliant up to this point but on this one occasion, I apparently was distracted. I hoisted his little body up on the seat like always and was waiting for him to finish.

All of a sudden he yells out, "Nana, you did it wrong! You have to point my doodle down!"

Sure enough, he had squirted between the little portable seat and the regular toilet seat. His little underwear and pants were soaked. Nana learned a valuable lesson that day. Always make sure to point the doodle down!

Now for the "booty" call.

In my grandchildren's vocabulary, what some of us call our tushy or behind, they call their booty. One day after taking one of the granddaughters to the potty, she informed me that I had to check her booty because sometimes she doesn't wipe well. She proceeded to explain to me that when that happens, it makes her booty hurt. This made sense.

Now, after a potty run, we always wait for the booty call which means, "Somebody come and wipe me!"

While visiting our home on another occasion, this same granddaughter had to use the potty. I waited for the booty call, having reminded her, right before she closed the door to the bathroom, to let me know when she needed help.

But there was no call for help.

After a little while my granddaughter came strutting out of the bathroom as if all was normal. I told her I needed to check her booty to make sure everything was clean. Back into the bathroom we went.

She was way too compliant, and I should have been suspicious immediately.

As I thought about it later, it was pretty remarkable that she willingly went back to the scene of the crime. While in the bathroom, doing the booty check, I glanced over and noticed that the water in the toilet was up to the rim. Not a good sign.

After examining the toilet paper roll I came to realize that about half a roll of paper was gone. I asked my granddaughter if she had put all that paper in the toilet. She calmly confessed that she had.

I then sent The Grand out of the room with a stern scolding and went to work trying to unstop the toilet. After several unsuccessful attempts with the dreaded plunger, I gave up. I decided to wait for my husband to get home from work. Just what a man wants to hear when he comes through the door. Right?

After arriving home, Russell shed his jacket, rolled up his sleeves and went to work. His first attempts were not successful either. This job called for backup so out comes the snake, a long, flexible tool that you maneuver through plumbing pipes. While my hubby loves it when he gets to use a tool, this one is not a favorite for obvious reasons.

Two hours later still no flush.

Just when Russell was about to concede defeat, he tried one more time and woo hoo, the big flush! Needless to say, this granddaughter was not allowed to go to the potty without supervision for quite a while after that incident. In addition, my toilet is now scarred for life. The snake left permanent scratches all over the bottom of my formerly pristine white ceramic toilet.

This is not the first time that child has left permanent damage on something. I doubt it will be the last. She's just that kind of kid!

Sometimes You Just Can't Put the Doodle Down

During one of the many visits from The Grands, all of the family decided to take a walk down by the creek near our house. As is the norm when you have preschoolers present, we make sure that all the kids use the potty before we leave. If we don't, one of them will inevitably need to go.

On this particular outing, one of our grandsons was being

particularly obstinate about everything that day. Going to the potty was no exception. As it so happens, Pop doesn't have much patience for three-year-old tantrums, so he decided to handle the situation. He escorts the grandson screaming and bawling into the bathroom. Pop proceeds to set him on the potty seat, tells him to point his doodle down, and finish so we could go for our walk.

Our grandson replied in a very tearful state, "I caaaaan't put my doodle down 'cause I'm cryyyyyyyyyyying!"

Apparently when one has his head thrown back and his tear-filled eyes closed, it is not conducive to getting the job done properly. Eventually, everything came out okay, and we all enjoyed our walk.

The Flush

The same precocious child in the booty story also has a knack for throwing things down the toilet and watching them flush. Nothing is sacred. In addition to the paper incident that nearly flooded our bathroom, this little adventurer has sent many an item down the same watery path.

For the sake of continued anonymity in this chapter, I will refer to her as Little One. Here are just a few examples:

Panties: During the potty training days Little One didn't want to wear big girl panties. She preferred her pull-ups. I imagine it was a security thing. If she had an accident there would be no mess.

On this particular day, much to her dismay, Little One

wasn't given a choice. She had to wear the dreaded panties. Later, while having some potty time, she decided the undies had to go. When her daddy turned his back to her—Mistake #1—she picked the panties up and tossed them into the toilet. Super-fast daddy fishes them out of the toilet water and tosses the dripping garment into the nearby tub. He explains to Little One that panties do not go into the potty.

As daddy turned away yet again—Mistake #2—Little One snags the panties from the tub and pushes the lever to flush the potty. Without so much as batting an eye, she drops the panties into the toilet and down they go, never to be seen again.

I did not dare to ask what happened to Little One's backside. Nanas do not want to know when their darlings must be chastised, even when it is warranted.

Toothbrush: Our middle granddaughter was sitting on the potty doing her business when Little One decided her sister was taking way too long. In protest, she threw her sister's toothbrush into the toilet water. That was bad enough, but there was also poo in there.

However, on a positive note, at least the toothbrush didn't get flushed. So who fished it out? Mama saved that one for Daddy. Isn't she nice?

Jewelry Cleaner: Little One decided the toilet water needed some sprucing up. Somehow she managed to get her hands on a container of jewelry cleaner her mother had recently used.

You know where this is going.

She poured the entire contents, jar and all, into the toilet. The water was a pretty shade of blue and, fortunately, the container was saved from the now infamous flush.

Unfortunately, there are a few more items that failed to escape the Little One's fascination with flushing. There were containers of salves and creams, miscellaneous small toys, socks, and an empty toothpaste tube. The tube was empty because Little One had taken the liberty of squeezing its contents into the toilet first.

By now, I am sure, you are thinking, why in the world do these people let that child be in a bathroom on her own?

Believe it or not, often times there was an adult right there with her. You turn your back for a second and in a twinkling of her mischievous eyes, the deed is done. I'm impressed that the plumbing in their home still functions.

I am happy to report that Little One has graduated to other adventures in the bathroom besides flushing. After she got older, there was a period of time where she insisted she needed her privacy. Big mistake. While left unattended in the bathroom, she managed to do some unbelievable things.

One day, Little One felt the need for a sink bath. With the door closed and her mother oblivious, the adventure began. Somehow she managed to find a small plastic tub, climbed upon a little footstool, and put the tub in the small vanity sink.

Now picture this. A small sink, an even smaller plastic vessel and a little bit of cold water. Add a very petite three-year-old and you have the perfect storm.

I don't know how she managed to fit into the small plastic tub, especially while having to avoid the faucet. Let's just say this is one determined kid.

By this time, I had arrived for a visit, and her mother asked me to check on her. As I opened the door, I couldn't believe the scene before me. Not only was the little sprite sitting in a tub of water inside the sink, she was washing herself with liquid soap and her toothbrush.

When I could finally speak, I asked her what in the world was she doing.

"I needed to wash some dirt off," she replied in a very matter-of-fact tone. She then looked at me like I was the one with the problem.

God help us all.

Little One is now at the four-year-old mark and she has become less adventuresome, at least in the bathroom. However, if after a few minutes alone she doesn't emerge, an adult is off and running.

Shooo, Maggie Smells!

As you may recall, I'm not naming names, however, this Grand never ceases to amaze me. She has the unabashed ability to come up with the darnedest things to do and say.

I have yet to introduce you to our "granddog." She is a beautiful chocolate and white Springer Spaniel. Her name is Maggie, although, Lady Margaret of Sheffield is her legal name. She was a wedding present from my daughter to her soon-to-be husband.

Maggie has been a great dog for this family and The Grands absolutely love her. They kiss and hug on her all the time. The girls even put dress-up clothes on the poor thing. Additionally, Maggie is allowed to go on camping trips with the family.

She is one lucky canine.

On one particular day when I was "Grand" sitting, Maggie lay sprawled out on the floor of the family room. For reasons I can't even begin to explain, one of The Grands decided to bend over and sniff the sleeping dog's booty. The child then loudly proclaims, "Shoo, Maggie smells bad!"

In instances like this, I really do try to downplay the behavior. I calmly said to the child, "Well, perhaps you shouldn't be sniffing her booty."

Later when her mother returned I told her what had transpired. She wasn't the least bit surprised. Mama merely stated in a very nonchalant voice, "Oh yeah, that's her [the Grand's] new thing. She goes through the house, walking behind Maggie and sniffing her booty."

Oh good grief. I'm beginning to think counseling may be in this child's future.

Poo at the Mall

Because I need backup to tell this unbelievable story, it is impossible for the subjects to remain completely anonymous. Sorry.

Jenny often takes my three granddaughters to the local shopping mall. For one thing, they love to shop—I wonder where they get that obsession?—and two, in the summer months they run out of things to do. The shopping mall is cheap entertainment. The twenty-five-cent rides and a cookie or ice cream cone helps ward off the boredom.

However, The Grands' favorite thing to do at the mall is to meet Nana. They usually try to persuade me to buy them something they just can't live without.

Like a good Nana, I often meet them at the mall. With three children under the age of six, backup for Jenny is quite necessary for obvious reasons. My daughter has an insatiable shoe habit and she can't always control the urge. On this particular trip, she decided to go solo.

Now, because I can't bear for you to miss one little detail of this hilarious story, I have asked Jenny to share it with you in her own words. Keep in mind the scene: a large shopping mall, one mother and three little girls.

The Little One, as Nana likes to call her, is into her third or fourth month of potty training. This third child of mine is stubborn, hard headed and fearless. She makes me question my parenting skills on an hourly basis.

We are shopping in my very favorite shoe department and there is a rest room not twenty feet away. Both Big Girls have already been to the potty, on two separate trips, mind you, because we wouldn't want to be logical and all go at the same time.

I try to entice, bribe and threaten the Little One into going both times but no dice. Her pull-up is dry and she isn't budging.

Okay, so I am now trying on some seriously cute strappy

sandals all the while trying to keep the girls from crawling on and under the shoe display tables. Alas, my last nerve is shot and I announce we are leaving the mall. Like right now!

The girls do not want to leave. They are crying and carrying on, and then I realize that Little One is under a shoe table. I have to crawl under the display to retrieve her.

Oh, my gosh. I smelled poo!

"You have got to be kidding me. Did you poop in your pants?'"

Her reply: "Um. No.'"

I pull up her dress, do the age-old diaper check, and yes, she had in fact pooped in her pants.

Now blame it on the fact that we've been potty training for a quarter of the year, or that I had a brain fade, or that I just pulled a rookie mistake. Whichever it was, I did not have the diaper bag with me. It was in the car at the opposite end of the mall. Of course.

We are about half way through the mall when I notice the Little One is waddling like a penguin. I'll admit, I am impatient and unsympathetic to my wee small girl, so I am not inclined to carry her. Instead, I practically drag her down the corridor of the mall.

We walk maybe ten feet more when she stops.

I look down and there is poop on the floor! The Big Girls follow my gaze and are saying, "Oooooh, Yuck!"

My darling girl, who had held it in for so long out of sheer obstinacy, had let the floodgates go. She is so thoroughly soaked, her pull-up is hanging down to her knees. Thus the penguin walk. Thus the poop falling on the mall floor.

I am mortified. Totally, completely, utterly and wholeheartedly mortified.

I quickly look around to see if I've been identified as the worst mother on the planet. Fortunately, no one seems to notice that I'm standing over something very suspicious looking.

Hurriedly, I shush my Big Girls, threatening their lives if they so much as utter a word that would call attention to us. I grab one of the two tissues in my purse, pick up the poop and in a mad dash, run to the nearest trash can. I return to the scene of the crime, squirt hand sanitizer on the floor, and use my one remaining tissue to give the floor a quick swipe.

Next I swoop a completely unaffected Little One up in my arms and we all hightail it all the way back to my car. I mean, I am knees-to-chest moving through that mall.

Thank goodness I didn't run into anyone I knew. To this day I still can't look at that particular spot of floor at the mall without breaking into a flop sweat at the memory.

I'm sorry I missed that little adventure.
Well, maybe I'm not.

> *When I woke up this morning I had one nerve left. Danged if you ain't got on it!*
>
> - Anonymous

Chapter Five
Holiday Hoopla

The holidays are so special to me, and even more so since The Grands have come along. They bring such an innocent wide-eyed wonder to all that is magical about this time of year. The presence of grandchildren in my life takes me back to wonderful memories I have of holidays long ago.

My family would travel to my Granny's house every Christmas Eve. A large, extended family gathered there in her quaint little home to celebrate the season. One of my favorite memories is that of Granny telling us the story, The Night Before Christmas. She didn't have a copy of the book; she always told it from memory. We would often ask her to tell it over and over.

If I close my eyes I can still hear her sweet voice saying, "Twas the night before Christmas, when all through the house…"

After my siblings and I grew up and started having families of our own, we moved the tradition of gathering our family to my parent's home. I have three brothers and two sisters. Between us there were eleven grandchildren and later a few great-grandchildren. Throw in a few aunts, uncles and cousins and it was utter chaos. There were so many people it was hard to move from room to room.

Everyone brought token gifts and, by the time they were placed around the small tree in the living room, you could barely see the floor. Dad observed it all from his comfy recliner while trying to listen to Christmas carols on his stereo. I think he loved Christmas almost as much as I did. Mom would pace from the living room to the back of the house where the kitchen was. All the commotion made her very anxious. I don't know how she survived six kids.

Typical of holiday gatherings, we always had lots of food at my parents' Christmas Eve celebration. There was always peppermint and horehound stick candy along with unshelled walnuts and pecans. The nuts were held in a large wooden bowl with a nutcracker tucked among them. Other favorites included chocolate fudge, fruit cake, and the proverbial cheese and cracker tray.

However, it was the large red glass punch bowl with red punch in it that was the highlight of the celebration. That punch bowl became our family tradition. It was always placed at the end of the island counter top within easy reach of all. The younger kids would argue about who would help my daddy prepare the punch each year. It was an honor and a privilege.

The Red Punch Bowl never missed a Christmas Eve at my parent's house.

After both parents passed away and their house was sold, there was some confusion about which one of the six grown children had possession of The Red Punch Bowl. None of us had any recollection of what happened to it. Had it been boxed up with the donated items when we cleaned out the house? Needless to say, we were heartbroken.

The first Christmas without either of my parents rolled around. We missed them so much. It was even more difficult because we weren't gathering at our family home. However, we were determined to keep the tradition of gathering our families together on Christmas Eve.

It was decided that my oldest sister, Joy, would host our holiday celebration at her home. Bittersweet as it was, we all filed in with our peppermint and horehound candy, chocolate fudge and cheese trays. I am happy to say there was no fruitcake.

As I entered the dining area of my sister's home and glanced at the kitchen counter, there it was. The Red Punch Bowl with red punch in it. Apparently, my younger sister Gay had it all this time and just didn't realize it. She found it just before the holidays and decided to keep it as a surprise for all of us.

It was our Christmas miracle that year. The Red Punch Bowl continues to grace our celebration, no matter whose home we bring the holiday chaos into.

The takeaway from this story is this: make memories with your grandchildren. You never know which memory they will tuck away in their heart only to bring it out again one day to share with their own children and grandchildren.

The Unconventional Nativity

It is important to me that The Grands understand the true meaning of Christmas. They have been taught that it is a celebration of the birth of Jesus Christ and they embrace that. We have many picture books about the very first Christmas, and they love having these read to them. We also put a Happy Birthday Jesus decoration on their Christmas tree, located in the playroom at our house.

Even at their young age they have been able to keep commercialism of the holiday season in perspective for the most part.

One afternoon, after four-year-old Greer had stayed at our house, I went up to the playroom to pick up any toys left out and to check on things. I have learned to do this because I almost always find something unexpected that the creative little minds have decided to do while under limited supervision. I was not disappointed.

The first thing I noticed was the child-sized plastic nativity set, which was placed under their decorated tree, was missing some pieces. In fact, all of the main characters were gone. The only thing left was the actual manger, a palm tree and a bale of hay. Even the angel who was usually perched on top of the manger was missing.

As I began to look around the room and check out what I thought might be a logical place to relocate a nativity scene—the bookshelves, toy box or closest—I was both surprised and delighted at what I discovered.

Greer had apparently decided the manger was a bit

outdated and wanted to provide a more comfy place for baby Jesus to make His entrance. She had, in fact, relocated them all to the two story doll house. There, in the living area, was the whole gang. Mary and Joseph were on the sofa along with one of the sheep. A shepherd was lounging in a puffy chair with the donkey standing at his side. Baby Jesus was tucked nicely in a blanket on top of the cocktail table, which was placed in the middle of the room.

Greer didn't leave anyone out. The wise men were lined up outside the front door, waiting to get in to see the new arrival. They weren't alone. Evidently Noah, his wife and sons, along with two of every kind of animal on earth decided to pay their respects to the newborn King.

As for the missing angel, she was perched on top of the two story doll house. Someone had to keep watch over the blessed event.

Santa Figured Out

Our eight-year-old granddaughter, Allie, is at that age where she has been struggling with whether to believe in Santa. I think she understands that in reality, he is fictitious. However, in her heart I think she secretly hopes he is real. I know a lot of her friends are starting to question Santa's existence as well.

Allie is very is torn, or so I thought.

A few weeks prior to Christmas we were together, talking about the ingenious and very popular elf toy that is now all the rage. Parents move the toy to different locations in the home throughout the holiday season. Children are told the elf keeps an eye on them—taking note if they have been a good or bad—and then reports back to Santa each evening.

Allie's two younger sisters are die-hard believers in both Santa and the "spy" elf, and I could tell Allie had been giving this a lot of thought.

She looked at me and said, "Nana, I don't think that elves make our toys. I believe Santa just goes to the toy store and buys them." Before I could recover enough to answer, she blurts out, "Oh yeah, and Santa's a stalker too. He watches people while they sleep."

I can't imagine where kids come up with this stuff. I don't know if growing up is harder on The Grands or on me.

Is There an Elf in the House?

Did I mention that I love Christmas? During the holiday season, my house reflects this, much to the dismay of my husband. Russell tells me I have an illness. I decorate every nook and cranny in the house. I use the excuse that it's for the grandchildren. Although, I have to say, they do seem to appreciate the days and days it takes to put up all the decorations.

The Grands would be terribly disappointed if I didn't put a tree up in their playroom or the mini tree in their bathroom or the trees in the bedrooms or the tree in the family room. You get the picture.

In their playroom room I admit I go overboard on the decorations. It's just that I want them to experience all the magic that the holidays bring. To me, that means surrounding yourself with things only brought out once a year. For instance, their tree is adorned with all the things they aren't allowed to enjoy very often—cupcakes, ice cream cones, lifesaver garlands, hard candy spirals and gum balls. The Grands shared with me that Baby Jesus probably liked all these goodies too.

The tree also holds ornaments celebrating their very first Christmas. Each ornament was made special by adding their name and birth date. The Grands love that they get to put their ornament anywhere on the tree they choose. We are making memories.

~♥~

Unfortunately, my grandsons do not live in our state. Because of that and the fact I have to share custody with the other set of grandparents, they only get to spend actual Christmas Day with us every other year. This past year, they came to town several days after Christmas.

Because I go all out to make their time with us special and memory-filled, I leave every bit of the decorations up. It thrills me to see their faces when they come into the house. Trees and garlands and lights, oh my!

On the day my grandsons arrived for their holiday visit, Sawyer, who was six at the time, ran up the stairs to the playroom to check out the tree. When he came back down he made a bee-line for me.

With a very concerned look on his face he stared me straight in the eyes and said, "Nana, why is that elf still here?"

Keep in mind this was several days after Christmas. The elf he was referring to was a small, decorative elf that I had placed on the table near his bunk. It faced the place Sawyer would lay his head at night.

At first, I didn't understand why the presence of the elf brought him such concern. Then it came to me. My decorative elf looked very much like the spying elf toy that was supposed to report a child's good or bad behavior to Santa. Sawyer was familiar with the spy elf because one had shown up day after day in his home before the holidays. It had even followed him across two states to South Carolina where he spent Christmas Day. According to his parents, the presence of the spy elf had kept Sawyer from doing many of the things he would have otherwise done—picking on his little brother, not eating his vegetables, talking too much in school, just to name a few.

I could see Sawyer's questions reflected in his eyes. Didn't all the elves return to the North Pole on Christmas Eve? Hadn't I made the good boy list? Why was that elf still in Nana's house? If that elf is still here, am I going to have to keep being good?"

Realizing the seriousness of the situation, I explained that my elf did not have the magical powers of the spying version. Sawyer seemed to find comfort knowing that the elf in his room upstairs had been a part of my decorations for many years.

Problem solved, or so I thought.

~♥~

In addition to the spy elf look-alike, I have some much larger elves that I acquired several years ago. While the small elves are only about six inches tall, the larger ones are closer to thirty inches in height.

These elves are among my favorites. How they came to live with me is a story in itself. I first saw them atop a tree in a wonderful inn located in the North Carolina mountains.

I probably would not have noticed them except there was a grown man, being instructed by his very determined wife, standing in a rocking chair looking up into a very tall decorated Christmas tree.

The wife was apparently looking for the brand of a very cute elf planted in the tree. The husband was attempting to read the name on the tag attached to the elf. The problem was, the elf was too high in the tree for the tag to be legible. The couple finally gave up and went on their dejected way.

Meanwhile, I was also very curious about these elves. They were quite whimsical with winking eyes, rose-colored cheeks and they had flexible arms and legs so you could pose them in any position. I thought if those elves are getting the kind of attention that warrants a grown man teetering on the edge of a rocking chair, they certainly needed a closer look.

Being a logical and somewhat sane person, I knew better than to stand on a rocking chair. With my luck, I would have splattered on the floor in a matter of seconds. However, I was not to be defeated. I too, wanted to know where those must-have elves came from.

As luck would have it, I just happened to have my small digital camera in my purse, so I proceeded to take a picture of the elf in the tree. Sure enough, once home, I enlarged the picture on my computer and that enabled me to make out the name of the manufacturer on the tag.

Persistence paid off and I am now the proud owner of not one, but four of the little darlings.

As part of my holiday décor, I posed one of the large elves on the newel post of my stairs. This way it appears he is greeting each of my guests as they enter. Another elf is perched on the rail at the top of the stairs looking down and waving. There are two more nestled in my family room tree. These are the elves my grandson had now come face to face with.

A few more days passed and we enjoyed a wonderful Christmas celebration with my daughter and her family. The boys had played with their cousins and their new toys. Finally, the after-the-holidays calm was settling in. We were making memories, I thought.

Then, without notice, my holiday bliss was shattered. Out of the blue, Sawyer came bounding into the room where I sat. He looked almost agitated. When I asked him what was wrong, he sternly replied, "Nana, those elves are freakin' me out!"

I suppose it is time rethink some of my holiday décor. My intent was to instill warm and fuzzy memories in my grandchildren, not give them nightmares!

Not Everyone Loves Santa

It is quite obvious now that Sawyer doesn't like the elves. I have also discovered that our middle granddaughter, Chase, is terrified of Santa. It is okay seeing him at the mall as long as Old Saint Nick keeps his distance, and she doesn't mind watching cartoons or movies with him as the star. What she does mind, however, is that he comes into their home on Christmas Eve.

Chase was so frightened last Christmas that her parents found her crying and trembling in her bed, long after her sisters were sound asleep. She didn't want Santa coming into their house.

Think about it. Our children are taught to stay away from strangers and never get into a car with one. And yet, we have introduced the image of a very large man in a bright red suit and lots of hair covering most of his face coming into Chase's safe place. We even feed him cookies for goodness sakes!

Well, Chase was not having any of it, and she was truly terrified. There was only one way her parents were able to get her to relax enough to go to sleep that night. They wrote a note to Santa, asking him to please leave the presents on their porch instead of coming down the chimney and into their home. This solution satisfied Chase, and she was able to then go to sleep.

~♥~

The problem of the jolly old stranger in the house has been resolved, but only temporarily. My guess is, this whole scenario will be repeated again next year. No one has asked, but here is my two cents on the subject.

If a child is that traumatized by the thought of anyone coming in the night, into a place that is their sanctuary, maybe it's time to tell them the truth. However, there is another solution right under the noses of my daughter and son-in-law. It is the twenty-five pounds of mischief living under the same roof. Read on.

Chase not only is afraid of Santa, but also the Tooth Fairy. She hasn't lost any teeth at this point but her older sister, Allie, was about to lose her first one. The tooth was very loose so her daddy decided it was necessary to pull Allie's tooth that evening. He was concerned it might come out while she was sleeping. While daddy pulled on the tooth one way, Allie jerked her head in the opposite direction.

The result was the tooth came out, went flying across the room, and was never found.

Allie was very concerned that the missing tooth meant that she would not receive a visit from the Tooth Fairy. The decision was made to leave a note explaining that it was Daddy's fault there was no tooth under the pillow. Could she, the Tooth Fairy, please leave the money anyway?

Allie was content with this solution, and she finally drifted off into peaceful slumber.

As it turned out, though, not everyone was at peace. In the middle of the night Jenny and Bradley were awakened by sobbing coming from the girls' room.

It was Chase. She was terrified that the Tooth Fairy was not only going to be in their house but also in her room. Before Jenny could get out of bed and get to Chase, she heard Allie yell out.

"Chase, it's okay. The Tooth Fairy has already been here!"

As Chase wiped her tears, Allie sat in the bed and proudly waved her dollar bill.

The next day their grandfather, Pop, was talking to three-year-old Greer about the Tooth Fairy incident. He asked her, "Greer, what would you do if you woke up and found the Tooth Fairy in your room?"

Without hesitation, Greer said, "I would just punch her in the nose!"

I think we need for Greer to take care of Santa while she's at it.

The List

As you have, by now, come to understand, I truly have a passion for the holidays. This passion is mostly because I have the great pleasure of watching my grandchildren observe this most wonderful time of the year.

They are at the perfect age of innocence. They believe.

Like all children, they get caught up in the excitement of all the festivities and wonderment that the holidays bring. You can see it in their twinkling eyes as they witness the magic of the season. However, on the other side of that twinkle, they are children after all. They fall prey to all the must-have toys that are advertised. They also still believe, thank goodness, that they have to behave if they want to receive the toys and other stuff on their wish list.

A few years ago my daughter Kristy and son-in-law Brant came up with a solution to the "gotta-haves" that I think is brilliant. Like most young children, our grandson Sawyer wanted every toy and gadget that was promoted on the Cartoon Channel. When he was old enough to understand, his parents explained to him about gift giving to others. They also told Sawyer all about Santa and the elves at the North Pole. He was all in at this point.

Kristy and Brant went further and explained all about The List that Santa keeps for all good little boys and girls. According to them, this is how The List works. Each time Sawyer asked for some toy he saw on television, his parents agreed to add it to The List. They further explained that when Christmas time came in December, Santa would determine which items on The List Sawyer would receive. This is, of course, based on how naughty or nice my grandson had been.

I'm telling you, Sawyer bought into this hook, line and sinker. This solution worked every time they entered a store selling all the things that little boys just had to have. In the days before The List, Sawyer would wander down each aisle of the store and ask for this or for that. More than once, he would throw a fit if he didn't get it. But now, since the introduction of The List, he calmly tells his mom or dad, "Put that on The List."

This works great, not just at Christmas time, but for birthdays and other occasions too. And, best of all, no more tantrums in the stores.

Now this concept has been working very well for several years. Then, one day, Pop decided to interject his mischievous sense of humor. While on a shopping trip with Nana and Pop, Sawyer found something he really wanted. He politely asked if we would tell his parents to put it on The List.

We agreed to do so, but then Pop decided he would have a little fun with Sawyer. He asked to see the infamous list. Our grandson did not hesitate one bit.

In his matter-of-fact way, Sawyer said, "Don't be silly Pop, The List is invisible. Santa is the only person who can read it."

Sometimes it's just hard to outsmart a six-year-old.

Something magical happens when parents turn into grandparents. Their attitude changes from "money doesn't grow on trees" to spending it like it does.

— Paul Lindon

Chapter Six
Sometimes It Just Hurts

A Sick Little Boy

I have already shared with you the experience our family had when little Greer spent time in the neonatal intensive care unit at our local children's hospital. There was another hospital experience with The Grands, this time with our second grandson Cohen when he was only seven weeks old.

It was just after Christmas when his family came to visit.

Because Cohen was born just before Thanksgiving, it was the first time most of our family had seen him. It was also in the middle of flu season. His parents, Kristy and Brant, were very careful to keep Cohen isolated as much as possible during that time.

Brant left early in the day on New Year's Eve to return to Georgia and his job. However, Kristy and the boys stayed behind to spend a few more days with Nana and Pop.

Now, there it was, New Year's Day, and we were thoroughly enjoying the visit. Everything seemed fine until I noticed Cohen didn't want to take his bottle. Not only was he not eating, he seemed lethargic and slightly warm.

I became concerned enough that I began patting the bottom of his feet in an attempt to wake him. I also placed a cool wash cloth on his face. No response.

Kristy decided to call her pediatrician, who in turn, instructed her to take Cohen to the hospital.

When we arrived and went through triage, they immediately gave him something to reduce the fever.

The waiting area was packed. I was concerned we would be sitting in the waiting room with a lot of other sick children for a long time. That would not be the case. The staff wasted no time in getting all of us into a room. They explained that they do not take any chances with an infant less than eight weeks old.

Cohen looked terrible. His skin was splotchy and he wouldn't wake up. Kristy was beside herself.

They quickly had a doctor come in, and she explained the need to do blood work to check for RSV and other things. RSV is a very serious respiratory virus that can sometimes be fatal, especially in newborns. They would also need to do a spinal tap to check for meningitis, another potentially fatal illness in young children.

Fortunately, the staff insisted we go out into the waiting area while they performed the necessary tests. I was thankful we were spared having to witness this tiny little baby being poked and prodded.

As soon as we got outside Kristy phoned Brant. She explained what was going on and that Cohen would be admitted to the hospital. They suspected RSV, but wouldn't know for sure until a 48-hour culture was complete. My son-in-law, who had just left the day before, turned around and headed back to his son.

When Kristy and I were allowed into the exam room, a nurse had inserted an IV in Cohen's tiny arm. A splint was also added to keep his arm immobilized. He looked so pitiful.

By this time, Kristy was allowed to climb up on the gurney, and Cohen was placed in her arms. They stayed that way until a room was ready. By the time we reached the fourth floor Cohen was wheezing horribly, so an oxygen mask was placed over his pale little face. I have never felt so helpless in my life.

Brant arrived soon thereafter. Over the next two days he and Kristy kept vigil by their little boy's bed side. It broke my heart to watch. Finally, the cultures were complete and showed negative for RSV and pneumonia. The diagnosis was that Cohen had a serious respiratory infection.

After being discharged, Cohen was allowed to return to Georgia. At home he continued breathing treatments. He improved only to develop the actual RSV virus a few weeks later. He was a very sick little boy, but thankfully he recovered.

When your child or grandchildren are being little monsters, sometimes it helps to remember times like these, when they were so sick and vulnerable. It is a reminder you could have lost them. The misbehaving doesn't seem so bad then.

The Bully Hits Home

Even as I write this, I still can't believe that bullying has affected our family.

One evening while having a video chat with Kristy and

her family, I asked my grandson Sawyer how his day at school had been. He said something, but I couldn't quite understand what he was saying.

Later, on the phone, his mom told me what he was trying to tell us was that he had been bullied at school that day.

I was stunned. Sawyer is in the second grade and just shy of eight years old.

Kristy went on to explain that Sawyer was on the playground when a classmate approached him. The boy told Sawyer that he couldn't play in that part of the playground. Sawyer moved to another area to play. This same boy came up to Sawyer a second time. He again told Sawyer to move on, that he couldn't play there either.

Fortunately, Sawyer told a teacher on the playground what was going on, and it was dealt with. The teacher also contacted Kristy to share with her what had happened.

Later at home, she and Brant discussed the incident with Sawyer and assured him that he didn't do anything wrong, that he did the right thing letting a teacher know what had taken place. They also told Sawyer they were proud of how he handled the situation.

Even though this was a minor incident, it brought such sadness to my heart. My grandson is too young to be dealing with a bully. I wish I knew what the answer is to this growing problem in our society. Does the old adage "kill them with kindness" even work anymore?

Our granddaughter, Greer, had a similar incident while in

preschool. I had picked her up from school, and in the car she shared with me that a schoolmate had told her she didn't want to be friends with her anymore.

Greer asked me, "Nana, why would she say that to me?"

Good gracious, these are four-year-old children.

I replied in a voice that was calmer than I felt that I didn't know why the other girl didn't want to be friends. I told Greer that she was a wonderful little girl, that anyone would be lucky to have her as a friend.

Thankfully, Greer was satisfied with my comment. Frankly, I was a bit surprised that she didn't take a swing at the other girl. Maybe our little slugger is growing up. But oh, how it hurts when someone mistreats our babies.

When Things Just Don't Work Right

Our oldest granddaughter, Allie, is in the second grade. She is a very polite, caring and sensitive young lady. She has a quick wit as well. She loves to tell jokes and her laugh is heartwarming.

However, this school year has brought many challenges. It would take an entire book to detail her struggles both academically and physically. We have learned she has a form of dyslexia which has explained her difficulties with school work. It seems that the second grade level of academics brought this to the attention of both her teacher and her parents.

In the process of assessing the dyslexia, it was found that she also has some motor processing issues. I asked my daughter Jenny how in the world we missed these now obvious problems. Jenny simply explained they had just attributed it to clumsiness. And thinking back, we all did.

Allie seem to stumble over her own feet, fall down a lot and have trouble doing basic childhood things such as jumping rope.

As the school year progressed, getting help for Allie proved to be quite difficult. Even though she had been diagnosed by highly qualified professionals, it was determined by the public school system that she did not meet the criteria for special consideration for modification of her schoolwork. This was due to the requirements mandated by the state's curriculum counselors.

While her parents and the four grandparents grew increasingly concerned for her, Allie, thankfully, did not see herself as being disadvantaged. Even during all of the testing required for a proper diagnosis, she seemed to take it all in stride.

Allie still recognizes that some school work easily frustrates her at times. Regardless, she loves going to school every day and truly enjoys learning. And, as difficult as it is for her, she finds much joy in reading. In spite of these challenges, Allie has persevered, and we couldn't be more proud.

However, her parents had a tough decision to make. After many consultations and much prayer, they decided to place her in a private school. This school offers a program that would tailor her academic requirements to what she is capable of doing.

This was not an easy decision. Not only does it put a huge financial burden on this family of five, but it would likely cause emotional trauma for another member of their household.

Chase, only 16 months younger, is Allie's shadow. They have been almost like twins all of their lives. The two have shared a room from the time that Chase left the crib and—what I love most about them—they also share their thoughts and secrets with one another. Their mother told me that after they go to bed each night and the lights are turned off, she will hear them chatting up a storm. I often wonder what they talk about.

While having dinner at their home one evening, we found out at least one thing they share in the darkness of their room at bedtime.

Both sets of grandparents were seated at the table, along with the rest of the family. There were six adults and the three children. Chase was about three years old at the time. Before eating, the family says a prayer and, from time to time, the parents invite the little ones to pray. They usually take turns.

On that particular evening, Chase piped up and said that she wanted to say the prayer. As we all prepared for her usual, "God is great, God is good" prayer, we were stunned when Chase began to recite, verbatim, The Lord's Prayer. If you are not familiar with this particular prayer, understand that it is long and has a lot of complicated words. This prayer used to be taught in elementary schools, along with the Pledge of Allegiance.

While Chase struggled with the pronunciation of some of those big words, she didn't leave out any part of that prayer. When she finished, we were all just dumbstruck, sitting with our mouths open in amazement. Finally, I recovered enough to ask Chase where she had learned that prayer.

She very softly replied, "Allie taught me." Now keep in mind that Allie is not even five years old yet.

My heart, as well as that of every other adult at that table, just melted. We later learned that Allie had been taught the prayer in her preschool class at church. While they lay in the dark at night, she had taught the prayer to Chase. We discovered that Allie had also taught Chase the Pledge of Allegiance, among other things.

Perhaps Allie is going to be a teacher. We shall see.

~♥~

This fall the two girls will attend separate schools. While we do not know yet how the separation of Allie and Chase is going to work out, I do know that Chase is very worried about it—so worried in fact that she has consulted her precious Ducky.

Ducky is Chase's security blanket. Apparently, she has received some very good advice from Ducky. She appears to have come to terms with attending school without her sidekick.

Chase has wisely figured out that little Greer will soon be starting school. She will need to show her little sister the ropes, just as Allie had done for her a couple of years earlier. Sometimes children just have to work things out for themselves without us. Sad, but true.

~♥~

Unfortunately, Chase's brave new attitude did not last. The closer it got to the first day of school, the more upset she became. She did not want to go to her new school, especially without her sister.

Allie, on the other hand, was very excited about attending a new school and couldn't wait to get there. She was also pumped that she would be wearing a cute little uniform. No worries there.

As that first day of school arrived, Bradley, Chase's dad,

decided he would park the car near the school and walk her into the school. I'm sure this is discouraged by school officials, however, this dad was not going to abandon his little girl in her time of need. Even he was struggling, knowing how anxious Chase was.

With a heavy heart Bradley left the school and went back to his car.

A little later that morning, I received a text from Jenny. She said, "I feel like I'm gonna puke just worrying about my girls, especially Chase."

I replied like a good mother should. "Everything is going to be okay." I also told her I had prayed that God would send a special angel to watch over Chase and calm her fears.

Jenny then told me that she had held Chase in her arms and rocked her to sleep the night before. And, while doing so, she and Greer said prayers for Chase. I was already tearing up, picturing this sweet moment between a mother and her daughters, when something else Jenny said finished me off.

Five-year-old Greer had apparently also prayed, "Please let Chasey have a friend before lunch." And you know what? Chase did make a friend before lunch and her name was Lola. Her first day in a new school ended much better than it began.

That Had to Hurt

If you have little ones in your life then you have had to witness at one time or another one of them taking a tumble and hurting themselves. Unfortunately, I have had to watch on more than one occasion.

I have to say, I would rather someone torture me as to see one of The Grands get hurt.

There is a cocktail table in my home, and it is one of The Grands' favorite places to play. It has two drawers facing the sofa and it is filled with all sorts of fun things. There are gloves, beaded jewelry, earrings, cars, puzzles, cards and lots of other goodies.

When The Grands come into that room that is the first place they go. Sometimes they even find something new that Nana has added.

However, on one particular day, it wasn't such a fun place to be. Our youngest grandson Cohen was rough-housing with Pop on the sofa. And, as usual, in the blink of an eye, he fell sideways off of the sofa and hit his cheek on the corner of the table.

I heard the scream and came running. His mother was in the shower and did not hear the commotion.

Pop was cradling a sobbing Cohen in his arms and his look told me it was a bad hit. I finally got Cohen to let me take a look, and I honestly thought I would cry. He had a huge knot on his little cheek just below his eye.

It had already started to bruise and had a small amount of blood at the center. I knew how badly that had to hurt.

Immediately I went to the freezer and got a bag of peas and wrapped it in a soft towel. Cohen allowed me to lay it on his cheek while he continued to cling to his Pop.

Now came the hard part: telling his mother.

I went upstairs to explain what happened, and warned her it looked really awful. Even having been forewarned, her eyes filled with tears when she saw the horrible swelling on her little man's cheek.

As is the norm, after some much needed cuddle time with mommy, Cohen settled down. The grown-ups in the room, not so much.

I can tell you that he had a heck of a shiner for the next few days. He actually seemed proud of it.

~♥~

We had another incident with little Greer.

All of my grandchildren have been taught to hold the rail when using the staircase in our home. For the most part, they are really good about this. I have explained that if they stumbled or tripped, their hold on that rail would prevent them from falling.

Greer and I were starting down the stairs together, and I am right beside her. She was on the side with the rail, and I thought she had a hold on it. I think because I was right there with her, she felt it was unnecessary. Somehow she caught her foot on the carpeted portion of the treads and down she went, tumbling head first, down the stairs.

I reacted as quickly as I could and managed to grab one of her feet to stop her from continuing all the way to the bottom.

Greer was howling as I gathered her into my arms to calm her down. I think she was more scared than hurt.

I know it sure took a few years off of my life. My heart was pounding. You can only think of the "what ifs" when something like that happens.

Thank goodness Greer only had a few scrapes on her tummy and a red spot on her chin.

I am sorry she fell, but I can tell you she doesn't come down those stairs without holding the rail anymore, even if I am right beside her.

This spill was also a reminder of just how quickly something can happen. Sometimes we can prevent the accidents and sometimes we can't. We are not super heroes, even though The Grands think we are at times.

~♥~

This last incident happened just days before this manuscript was finalized. It was the most serious injury any of The Grands had suffered to date. It is also was one I hope is never repeated.

The injury happened to Cohen, our youngest grandson. Apparently he is going to be the one that makes emergency room trips with some regularity—no surprise really since he is also the most active one of the bunch. He knows only one speed: fast.

Once again our daughter Kristy and her three children were visiting for a few days while her husband was out-of-town. They were at the end of their stay, the van was packed, and they were ready for the return trip home. However, it was decided that all of us would meet Aunt Jenny and her girls for lunch before they left town.

We met at a casual dining restaurant and had a fun-filled lunch. Afterwards, everyone said their good-byes. Kristy, needing a dress for an upcoming wedding, asked me if I would accompany her and the kids to a department store that was located across the street from where we had eaten. I explained that I had another appointment, but I could spare about twenty minutes.

As we entered the store, I took the boys to the toy department. They immediately found a novelty drinking cup which I agreed to buy. Kristy with baby stroller in tow headed for the dress department. About twenty minutes later I took the boys to join their mother. I gave them money for their purchase and explained it was time for me to leave.

I felt bad leaving Kristy with three children while she was trying on clothes, and told her so. She assured me she could handle it, saying, "Mom, I do this all the time."

Apparently after I left, she indeed was able to try on dresses, make her selection, and head to the checkout line. By that time, I was well on my way to my appointment a half an hour away. I had just sat down in the waiting area when I received a call no one wants to receive.

It was Kristy.

"Mom, you have to leave right now and come help me! Cohen has fallen and he has to go the emergency room. The paramedics are here now. Jenny is on her way to get the other two kids." She told me what hospital they were headed to and hung up.

I explained to the receptionist my emergency and hurried out the door. Because I knew I was at least twenty-five minutes away, I called Pop to have him meet Kristy at the hospital. I had just hung up from talking to him when Kristy calls back.

"Mom, the paramedics have decided to take Cohen downtown to Children's Hospital instead of the one closer. I am in the ambulance with him. Just meet us there."

What? They are in an ambulance!

At this point I had no idea how Cohen got hurt, so I was

imagining the worst. Again, I called Pop to make him aware of the change in hospitals.

As it turned out, Pop arrived at the hospital ahead of the ambulance and was in the waiting room when Kristy and Cohen walked through the door. Cohen was thrilled to see a welcome face and ran straight into the arms of his grandfather.

Obviously, he did not have a life-threatening injury.

I arrived soon after, and it absolutely took my breath to see my three-and-a-half year old grandson sitting in a chair with a large bandage under his chin and blood all over him. Even Cohen's beloved "monkey" blanket Mo Mo, which he had a death grip on, had blood on his head and face.

Kristy did not look much better. She too had blood down the front of her shirt. But what really grabbed my heart was the small, bloody handprint on the top of her shoulder. Obviously, this had occurred when Cohen clung to his mommy after she picked him up.

Finally, I found out what had happened.

As Kristy and baby Piper waited in the checkout line to pay for her purchase, both boys were standing behind her. They were waiting their turn to pay for the drink cups I had given them money to buy. As I said earlier, Cohen is always in constant motion, and in his playful state he somehow managed to trip on the carpet. This caused him to pitch forward and fall onto the bottom of a clothing rack that had a square metal edge. The impact cut a one-and-a-half inch gash just below his jawbone.

You can just imagine the scream he let out.

When Kristy turned to see what had happened, there was blood gushing from the wound. Cohen tried to put his hand over it, only to cause a large amount of blood to run down his arm and all over his favorite super hero tee shirt.

Kristy immediately picked him up and ran to the checkout counter, seeking help. Fortunately, a family shopping nearby realized the seriousness of the situation and took charge of the other two children.

The department store personnel acted quickly. After dialing 9-1-1, they immediately began to pull clothing off a nearby rack. These were used as a compress in an effort to stop the bleeding.

When the paramedics and firemen arrived, they proceeded to lay Cohen flat, right there on the checkout counter. The emergency personnel continued to apply pressure to the wound.

By this time, additional store employees had returned from the housewares department with clean white towels that the paramedics had asked for. Eventually the bleeding slowed enough for them to place a bandage on the cut. Because there was concern that Cohen may have nicked an artery, the decision was made to take him to the hospital in the ambulance so that he could be attended to in the event the bleeding increased. Kristy readily agreed. She was an emotional wreck and couldn't imagine having to drive herself anywhere.

In the meantime, Jenny had arrived to find both an ambulance and a fire truck at the entrance to the department store. She had no idea what she and her three girls were walking into. They certainly weren't prepared for the scene I just described.

Sensing that eight-year-old Sawyer was probably traumatized by all that had happened, Jenny quickly gathered her nephew to her chest and gave him a big hug. She also thanked the family that had been watching Sawyer and Piper.

Kristy then asked Jenny to take the other two children home with her, but not before paying for the drinking cups that the boys wanted. She also needed to pay for the dress Kristy was attempting to purchase.

As it turned out, it wasn't necessary to pay for the cups. The family that was helping to watch Sawyer and Piper had already paid for them. In addition, the department store gave Kristy a really nice discount on the dress.

Jenny was now headed home with five kids, two novelty drinking cups and one greatly discounted new dress. Kristy and Cohen were on their way to the emergency room via ambulance.

After Cohen went through triage at the hospital and had the original bandage replaced with a gel pack, we waited to be called back to a treatment room. It was while in triage that Kristy got a really good look at Cohen's injury. Not only was it a large cut, it was deep. Fortunately the gel pack that was applied contained an analgesic to numb the area. This meant no needles and that was a very good thing.

When the time came, Kristy and I both were allowed to go into the treatment room with Cohen. For a child that is pretty hyper most of the time, I was surprised at how calm and compliant he was. Trauma will do that I suppose.

Another assessment was done by the physician's assistant to determine any artery involvement because the wound continued to bleed. There also was concern there could be nerve damage because his mouth on that side was drooping.

Knowing the time had come to close the wound, I was concerned about keeping Cohen still long enough for the procedure to be done. It turned out there was no need to worry at all.

A hospital staff member brought an iPad into the room and allowed Cohen to choose a cartoon to watch. With Cohen flat on his back and his head tilted back, the young lady held the iPad about eight inches from Cohen's little face and he didn't move at all. Approximately thirty minutes, seventeen stitches and a purple Popsicle later, it was over.

Cohen, along with his brother and three girl cousins, were really impressed with the size of his wound and the cool stitches just below his jawbone. He wore them like a badge of honor.

Fortunately, Cohen's adventure was over and he was as active as ever by the next day. Our little man now has a not-so-lovely scar that I'm sure will provide him with a great story that will impress many female admirers in his future.

~♥~

The Grands have had busted chins, fractured arms, scraped knees and lots of bruised shins. We can now add seventeen stitches to the mix. I'm sure there is more to come and our hearts will hurt with each new incident. Those kinds of hurts will heal. Our grandchildren are still quite young and with the exception of the bullying I mentioned earlier and the occasional tearful comment such as "she won't be my friend," they have yet to experience the kind of hurt that penetrates their soul.

Oh, how I dread that day for I know it will come.

It is a part of growing up that must be experienced. It is

also those situations that will help them become who they are meant to be. I pray that they are little hurts. After all, The Grands are my babies now and for always, and I want to protect their sweet little hearts forever. Sometimes it just hurts to think about it.

> *Grandparents are like a piece of string. Handy to have around and easily wrapped around the fingers of their grandchildren.*
>
> — Author Unknown

Chapter Seven
The Gift of Time and Making Memories

The addition of The Grands to our family has blessed my heart beyond measure. Each one is a precious gift that I will never take for granted.

Scripture tells us if we teach our children right from wrong according to biblical principles, they will not forget what they have been taught. It is a natural assumption that it would be the job of the parents to do the teaching, however, I strongly believe it is the responsibility of grandparents as well.

I once heard a grandparent proclaim, "I've raised my kids, and I'm not going to raise theirs." That makes me sad.

Instead, I believe in the saying, "Grandparents are as important to a child's growth as vitamins."

If necessary, I would raise any one of my six grandchildren. I just can't let Pop hear me say that. He might head for the hills!

The Grands come in sets of three. If I have to keep them

for more than two days at a time, I am utterly exhausted. I just don't have the stamina I used to.

My grandchildren don't understand why Nana doesn't jump rope anymore. It's because my joints hurt. Or, why I don't climb a tree with them. I just can't—or maybe I could but then I might not get down without the fire department being summoned!

The most uncomfortable situation I get myself in sometimes is when I sit on the floor with The Grands. For some reason these children like to play games that require rooting around on a rug. After just a few minutes, my hip joints lock up and I can't get up off the floor.

They think it's funny. But, I tell you, it hurts like the dickens.

Because none of The Grands are strong enough to pull me up, I have to get on all fours like a dog, then crawl until I find something to pull up on.

On occasion, one of the little ones will grab an arm or leg and try to help. By this time, the others are rolling on the floor laughing.

Fortunately, I have a sense of humor and am usually laughing with them. As a grandparent, you have to be able to laugh at yourself. Otherwise, you will never survive with your dignity intact.

It is also my belief that our time is the greatest gift we can give to our grandchildren. I have found that no matter what you do with them, it doesn't seem to matter. After all, we can do no wrong, right?

I get all warm and gushy when I walk into a room where one or more of The Grands are gathered. Without fail, they call out my name and rush across the room to jump into my waiting arms.

It doesn't get any better than that.

When I have The Grands over to my house, I like to make sure we do something fun. Sometimes it is as simple as getting out paper and crayons to draw pictures or make cards. Other times, we make popcorn and hot chocolate and watch a movie together. One of my personal favorites is making cookies. The kitchen is a disaster afterward but worth the mess.

Some of the best times though, are usually when something hasn't gone as planned. It is the mishaps that bring the most laughter and make the very best memory makers.

Pumpkins Anyone?

Each year, as the leaves begin to fall, Pop and I gather The Grands and take them to a local pumpkin patch. Sometimes we even let their parents tag along.

This has become such a wonderful tradition for us, and we always look forward to it with much anticipation.

The pumpkin patch we chose this past year was also a working farm. In addition to the pumpkin patch, we were delighted to find an array of farm animals happy to be admired—albeit from afar—by five little observers. There were chickens, goats, ducks, horses, a donkey, sheep and some piglets. Our eight-year-old granddaughter Allie took one look at the piglets and immediately began chanting, "Bacon…Bacon…Bacon."

I was glad the little piggy couldn't understand English.

As our family continued a tour of the farm, everyone became interested in watching a momma cow and her calf. They were in a fenced-in area adjacent to the barn.

The Grands were fascinated with these bovines. All five, ages three to almost eight, were lined up in a row, standing on a lower part of the fence. This allowed each of them to be able to peep over the top rail to take a closer look.

Everyone was having a great time until Allie of "Bacon… Bacon…Bacon" fame, slipped off the fence and startled the momma cow. The animal charged the fence in defense of her calf, scaring the living daylights out of five little bug-eyed kids. All The Grands let out a scream and scrambled off the fence as fast as their little legs would allow.

The poor calf was just about as traumatized as the kids.

Our day came to an end with each grandchild tromping through the pumpkin patch in search of the perfect pumpkin. The Grands were worn out and with their prizes in hand, we finally headed home. No doubt those little pumpkins found a special place outside each of their homes for all to see.

As for Nana and Pop, we didn't need a pumpkin outside our door to remind us of our trip to the pumpkin patch. We had some very special memories of time spent with our five grandchildren tucked away in our hearts.

Don't Forget the Lovies

Some of the best memories I have of my daughters are those of them with their Lovies—that's what our family calls the little blankets, stuffed animals or dolls that becomes security for our little ones.

Jenny had a small patchwork quilt and a Holly Hobbie miniature doll. By the time she had outgrown the quilt, it was in shreds and Holly Hobbie was missing one of her pigtails.

~♥~

Kristy's Lovies were two tiny little stuffed puppies. She would carry them around, one under each arm. When she was potty training, she would sit on one potty seat and the puppies would be in another potty beside her. They did everything together.

As Kristy grew older, her favorite Lovie became Doggy, a larger brown and white stuffed Beagle puppy. She received it as a gift from her daddy after minor surgery when she was thirteen months old. When Doggy had to be washed, it had to be done at night, after she went to sleep, then returned to her bed by morning. That stuffed puppy is in her room to this day.

On one occasion, Doggy got something sticky on him, so it was necessary he be washed during nap time. While the stuffed pup could be washed in a machine, he needed to be hung to dry. Our neighbor happen to have a clothes line so after a thorough washing, Doggy was pinned by his ears to the line outside. With luck, the sunshine would dry the puppy quickly so I could return him to Kristy's bed before he was missed.

Unfortunately, I wasn't lucky. Doggy wasn't dry by the time Kristy got up from her nap that day. She rose and, of course, immediately began looking for Doggy. She looked out the sliding glass door and spotted her precious Lovie hanging by his ears no less on the clothes line.

I attempted to explain that we were just waiting for him to dry, then she could have him back. But at eighteen months old, she couldn't understand the concept of waiting. Kristy stood at the door and cried over and over, "Doggy, Doggy."

It was quite pitiful to watch. Thankfully, it wasn't long before Doggy was back in Kristy's arms, and I had one happy little girl.

~♥~

Each of our Grand's have their own special Lovie. Because these objects become prized possessions, some very important lessons must be shared. Our family has learned by experience, and it is advice that every new parent or grandparent should heed.

When you pick out a Lovie for your child or grandchild, make sure you buy two!

There have been so many times Kristy and Jenny have had to resort to the backup. If you don't have a second Lovie, someone could be in for one very rough night. Also, this ensures that a Lovie is always available for nap time or other such emergencies in the event the other Lovie is in the laundry.

Another important fact that should be mentioned is that the two Lovies must be identical and equally used. This is so they look and feel exactly the same—very important!

Our first granddaughter Allie has a pink blanket with a bear head. She named it Hamie. We have no idea where the name came from.

Sadly, Hamie was once misplaced, and Allie wouldn't sleep without it. Jenny and I scoured the department stores looking for another blanket just like Hamie. Fortunately, we found one that was identical. Allie never knew the difference.

~♥~

Chase, the second of our granddaughters, was another matter. Her Lovie is a yellow mini blanket. And, it has a duck head at one corner. It was a gift that quickly became her favorite. His name is Ducky.

Having learned our lesson with Hamie, we tried to locate a second Ducky.

No luck. We searched every store in town. We also searched the internet. No Ducky! Therefore, we are very, very careful with Ducky. He is looking ragged and tired, but he is also very well loved.

Besides Allie, Ducky is Chase's only other confidant. She shared with me that she talks to her beloved Lovie about lots of things, especially when she is worried about something.

We just hope nothing ever happens to Ducky. Otherwise, Chase may never sleep through the night again!

~♥~

Sawyer has Gilly. It is a tiny, very soft blue blanket with satin binding. He also has Puppy, a small light brown stuffed dog he received as an infant. There is only one Puppy and one Gilly. These two Lovies are always with him, even when he travels to see both sets of grandparents in other states.

Sawyer shared with me once that Gilly and Puppy help

him feel better when he is sad or upset, and that they give him big hugs.

We did have one crisis with Gilly and Puppy, however. After Sawyer and his family left to return home after a visit with us, I discovered both Gilly and Puppy had been accidentally left behind. A big uh oh. I knew he would not sleep without them.

I quickly gathered them up and took them to the nearest shipping store. As soon as I entered the store with the blanket and puppy in hand, the clerk looked up and said, "Uh oh."

I replied, "Oh yeah. How quickly can I get these to South Carolina?"

Fortunately, Puppy and Gilly arrived safe and sound the very next day. However, there was a little boy far away who cried himself to sleep that lonely night. But what a reunion there was when that box arrived at Sawyer's house! He was one happy fellow.

~♥~

Mo Mo, Cohen's Lovie, was introduced to you in a previous story. This little brown blanket has a satin binding and a monkey head in one corner. And yes, we have two.

Cohen calls both of them Mo Mo. When he gets sleepy or is crying because he has gotten into trouble, it is Mo Mo to the rescue.

Because this strong-willed toddler gets into mischief a lot, I am sorry to say that Mo Mo has been taken away on occasion. This works better than any time-out chair ever did.

~♥~

As you now know, our little Greer had a really rough start. Many days in the neonatal intensive care unit at the children's hospital were cause for prayer requests among our family, friends and prayer groups.

In my bible study group, there was a precious woman named Marion. She was a delightful lady with sparkling blue eyes, and a smile that went on for days. Marion had a special ministry. She often provided little fluffy white stuffed lambs along with a lamb-related children's book to newborn babies or young children that were having a tough time.

When I arrived at class one day, Marion handed me a gift bag and said it was for Greer. It was one of the little stuffed lambs and the book. In a very short time, Greer became quite attached to this extremely soft and cuddly lamb.

Knowing it would please Marion, I took a picture of Greer holding the little lamb. It also showed how worn the tail was from where Greer had been chewing on it so much.

When I walked into class the following week, I gave Marion the picture. Without saying a word, she gave me that blazing smile of hers, turned, and picked up a gift bag from the floor. Handing the bag to me she said, "Oh, I have something for you too. I want you to have a lamb and a book to keep at your house. This way you can share them with your other grandchildren."

That was exactly the kind of gesture that Marion would often do. She was always thinking of others.

A few months later, I found out that our sweet Marion was very ill. As her illness progressed, some members of our bible study class, including myself, went to her home. We were there to decorate her Christmas tree. While there, I went into her kitchen and spotted something on her refrigerator that brought tears to my eyes. Among all of her family photos was the picture I had recently given her. There, looking back at me, was my grandbaby Greer, holding the lamb that Marion had given her. My heart could have burst with emotion.

It wasn't too long after that visit that our precious Marion passed away. At her memorial service, the pastor talked about Marion's ministry. Apparently, there were a lot of people, adults and children alike, who had received one of Marion's lambs. The pastor went on to say that if anyone in attendance was lucky enough to have received one of the lambs, then we were truly blessed. That's exactly how I felt, and I look forward to the day when I can share with Greer all about my friend Marion. She will then understand, even more, just how special her little lamb is.

Greer has named this sweet gift Lambie and they are inseparable. She also has two identical pink hippo blankets. Greer explains that the hippos are there so Lambie has someone to play with when she is not around.

Greer can be sweet when she wants to be.

Our newest granddaughter, Piper, is just now starting to need her Lovie. She has not one, but two, little pink blankets with lady bug heads.

To distinguish between which is the clean Lovie and which one needs to be in the laundry, Kristy came up with a great idea. She decided to have Piper's name embroidered on one, and her monogram on the other. Now we can tell them apart, something I wish we had thought of with the other grandchildren.

~♥~

Another observation I wish to share is never underestimate the power of the Lovie. Most children are very attached to these well-loved blankets and animals. They apparently bring them comfort and assurance in ways we can't begin to imagine.

As my grandchildren are beginning to outgrow their Lovies, my daughters and I have had a discussion about what to do with them.

Both Kristy and Jenny have keepsake boxes for each of their children. This is the place where all of The Grands' special mementos are stored including baby rattles, their first locks of hair, special handmade items and even their baby teeth. The Lovies will go in this keepsake box as well.

However, here are a few additional suggestions for Lovies. Place the Lovie in a shadow box. Another idea is to take a picture of the Lovie or, better yet, have an artist paint it. You could then frame it and hang it in the child's room. This way he or she can continue to keep it close by, even if they are too old to snuggle it.

What a special heirloom this would make for their future children.

~♥~

When I named this segment, Don't Forget the Lovies, my intention was to call attention to how special security blankets and other prized toys are to our precious grandchildren. Our family has discovered that there is something else you should never forget either.

Each time I am reminded of this particular event, I just have to laugh.

Kristy and the kids had come to visit, and it was the first time since Piper's birth. Normally, Kristy seems to bring half of her house during a visit, so when it is time to pack up for a trip home, it takes a while.

Finally, the day of this particular departure arrived, and Pop helped to get all of the luggage, bags, boxes, etc., into Kristy's van. Both boys were strapped into their car seats, and we had given all the hugs and kisses that would last until the next visit.

Kristy was about to get into the driver's seat when she turned for one last hug from Pop. She said, "Well, I hope I have everything, but I'm sure I have forgotten something. I always do."

The words had barely escaped her lips when her hand flew to her mouth. With wide eyes, she exclaimed, "I forgot the baby!"

We all had. Sure enough, she went back inside to retrieve the sweet bundle of joy snuggled up in her car seat sound asleep. We all had a good laugh over that, but I couldn't help wishing she had left her with us. I would have gotten to enjoy that sweetheart a little bit longer.

~ 💜 ~

I know it sounds awful that Kristy forgot to put the baby in the car but, in her defense, she was still getting used to having a third child to load up. I think this happens more times than you think. I remember a time during my childhood that something similar happened.

We had a large family that included my parents and six children. On Sundays, we often traveled across town to visit my Granny. All eight of us would pile into the family vehicle. Keep in mind cars had bench seats in those days and no seat belts required. The speed limit was much lower as well. That being said, you could put at least four of us in the back seat, one in the middle between my parents, and one of the smaller kids would lay behind the back seat in the window.

Crazy, I know. Today we would be hauled off to jail for such offense.

Well, on this particular Sunday visit, we arrived at my Granny's and everyone got out of the car. There were always lots of hugs and kisses with the greetings, and then my Granny asked where was my little sister Gay. Everyone began looking around the yard, the house and in the car. She was nowhere to be found.

Finally, it occurred to my parents that she had been left behind. A frantic call to our neighbors confirmed that she was indeed at home, safe and sound. My sister would stay at the neighbors' until our return home.

Needless to say, after that incident my parents counted heads before getting into the car. Not a bad idea, even today.

Outdoor Adventures

One of my favorite things to do with The Grands is to

take them for a walk. We have a lot of walking trails in our neighborhood and they are not too difficult for those with short little legs. It is such a wonderful opportunity to talk about all that God created for us to enjoy. I love the wonderment in their sweet little faces at even the smallest discovery.

In the fall when the leaves turn, the granddaughters like to gather all the brightly colored leaves into small bouquets. They pretend they are flower girls in a wedding. Don't you just love their imagination?

The boys always have to find just the right stick to use when they walk along the creek.

On our last visit, we were rewarded with a family of ducks bathing. Believe it or not, even Cohen sat still so as not to disturb their ritual. On one rare occasion The Grands were able to witness a beaver working on his new home along the creek bank.

Their favorite thing of all, however, was to toss small stones into the water and watch the ripples. The two boys especially liked to toss twigs into the water just to watch them drift downstream. This was so much better than watching TV or playing video games.

As we made our way back to the house, we had to cut through a small field. It was laden with yellow dandelions and another small purple flower that covered the ground. Cohen decided to gather a bouquet to bring home to his mother. He worked really hard picking the flowers and was rewarded accordingly.

The smile on Kristy's face let Cohen know it was very much appreciated.

Forever Memories

There are so many funny things that my grandchildren have done that bring laughter to my heart long after the event. Their antics have brought so much joy to my soul. Even when they are absent from me, the memories keep each one of them very near and dear to me.

As The Grands continue to grow, they exhibit more thoughtful habits that I have come to cherish even more. It is when I see them doing certain things, usually without being prompted, that I am assured we haven't done too bad a job in nurturing them. We, the parents and grandparents, are helping them to grow into caring human beings.

~♥~

One such forever memory occurred when I took Greer to lunch one day. It was just the two of us. This outing was a treat because usually either her mother or her two sisters would be with us.

Greer chose McDonald's. After we ordered our food and sat down, I reminded her we had to thank God for our food. As I prepared to say a prayer, she interrupted me and announced that she would like to do it.

As we bowed our heads I was prepared for one of Greer's usually quick prayers. Instead, she started singing, "God ouw Fadder, God ouw Fadder, we tank you, we tank you. For ouw many bwessings, for ouw many bwessings. Ahhmen. Ahhmen."

Greer was three years old at the time and couldn't pronounce "r" or "th" very well. However, that didn't keep her from singing her little prayer song at the top of her voice in the middle of a crowded restaurant.

I think some of us adults could take a lesson or two from Greer. My heart swelled a bazillion times that day.

~♥~

Allie recently celebrated her eighth birthday a few months ago. If you have children or grandchildren you probably understand how competitive birthday parties have become. It is insane. What happened to cake and ice cream with the family?

When Jenny asked her what she would like to do for her birthday, Allie didn't hesitate. She wanted to have a paint party with twelve of her friends. They would have pizza and a cookie cake to eat. It was decided that I would oversee the canvas painting, and the pizza and cookie cake was just a phone call away.

The party was a hit. Each guest painted a Christmas tree in the snow on small canvases. This was their party favor to take home.

And as for birthday presents for Allie, there wasn't any.

Allie had shared with her mother that instead of gifts for herself, she would ask her friends to bring new baby blankets. She wanted to donate the blankets to the neonatal intensive care unit at the local children's hospital. The party guests gladly did so.

A couple of days later Jenny and Allie, along with Allie's sisters and a family friend, took the blankets to the hospital. This wasn't a random act of kindness on her part. Not only did Allie remember that her youngest sister had spent time in the intensive care unit, but also that a very special family friend had spent months and months there. She knew how much the hospital had helped them, so she wanted to give back.

We were so proud of her.

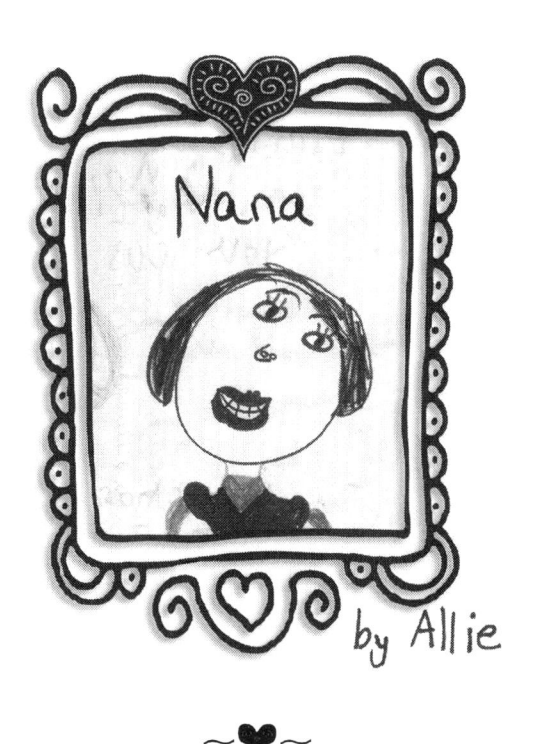

by Allie

I have already shared with you that we have a new granddaughter, Piper. She was born in the winter months and, because of the flu and RSV viruses that are prevalent that time of year, Kristy has been very careful to keep her away from just about everyone, at least for the first two months. My daughter explained to her boys that the reason Piper couldn't go to restaurants, shopping or to church was so she wouldn't get germs and become sick.

Sawyer pondered this. The next Sunday, while sitting in church with his father, the church pastor picked up the prayer requests that had been submitted that morning and began to share them with the congregation.

As he began to read one in particular, Sawyer just sat back and smiled.

"Please pray for my new baby sister so that she'll be healthy."

How sweet is that?

A grandmother was made to spoil you and save you from your parents.

– Author Unknown

Chapter Eight
Second Chances

It is my sincere belief that grandchildren are our chance at a do-over. I know without a doubt there are things I would do differently with my children if given the chance. There certainly are actions or words spoken that I regret may have influenced their lives.

As parents we have so much pressure and responsibility. Sometimes we miss something. Sometimes we just mess up. With our grandchildren, we don't have the same pressures we experienced as parents. That is what makes grandparenting so much fun, at least most of the time. However, I also believe it is still our responsibility to set an example of what a good person looks like.

Grandparents have the ability to influence the lives of our children's children. That is quite a task, but also it is an honor and one I look forward to. My hope is that I can be a positive role model for each of my grandchildren. I don't want to mess up these second chances that I have been given.

Like most grandparents, I absolutely love the time I spend with my grandchildren. It brings me more joy than I ever imagined.

The innocence is both refreshing and frightening. They are so vulnerable to our worldly influences.

My heart grows cold at the thought of what these precious souls will have to deal with in the not-so-distant future. Our modern culture sure isn't setting very good examples for them.

As difficult as it is to think about, I won't always be here for my grandchildren and, at some point, neither will their parents. I ask myself, what can I do? How can I, as a grandparent, help prepare The Grands for the future that is before them? What kind of legacy do I want to leave them?

The years are speeding by faster than I can stand. I wish I could push a pause button sometimes.

Recently, I have begun to have a sense of urgency about things that I want to experience with each of The Grands. Places to go, memories to share, things I want them to know. Mostly, I want them to understand that I will love them unconditionally and hug them to pieces every chance I get.

There are also important life lessons I want to help teach them. Here are a few that are close to my heart.

Help them to know God.

Teach them to pray.

Teach them to respect themselves and others.

Teach them to love one another.

Teach them to be kind.

Teach them to be responsible.

Teach them manners.

Teach them to have compassion for those in need.

Teach them to take care of themselves.

Teach them to look for the good in others, especially when it isn't obvious.

This, at times, seems to be an overwhelming task, but it's oh so important. Of course, as much as I like to think I am teaching The Grands all of these things, more often than not, they are teaching me so much more.

Funny how that works.

One last thing to think about. How often do we spend time with our children and our grandchildren?

I realize that some family members live away from us and it is difficult to see them often. However, in this day and age of social media, the possibilities are endless. My grandsons love having FaceTime with us. Video chats are the greatest thing since sliced bread.

Another issue, unfortunately, is just making time with family a priority. With our busy lifestyles, it is becoming more difficult to spend quality time with our loved ones.

If you are the matriarch or patriarch of your family, I encourage you to make gatherings a must. There is nothing better than a house full of people, Granny's chicken and dumplings, Aunt Helen's apple pie and lots of laughter.

Those Sunday dinners were the highlight of our week and some of my most precious memories. I was surrounded by my grandparents and a host of other family members.

Was it chaos? Yes. Was it difficult to do sometimes? Absolutely. But those gatherings at Granny's house were some of the best times of my childhood. I want the same experiences for The Grands.

It is memory-making times like this that are so important to the well-being of our grandchildren. They need to feel a part of something special. They need to know they belong.

Also, being a part of an extended family gives our grandchildren the assurance that someone will always be there for them. That is so important.

Families are all unique. Each is made up of different personalities, intellect and opinions. Some of us are sweet, kind and tender-hearted. Others may be rough, tough and hard-hearted. It is the mix of the good, the bad and the ugly that makes us family.

My daughter Jenny wrote the following poem years ago while in elementary school. I think it explains family dynamics much better than I could.

A Box of Crayons
By Jennifer Kelley Greer

My family is very expanded and different,
So my family is like a box of crayons.

Some are short
Some are long
Some are fat
Some are thin
Some aren't wrapped well
Some are broken
Some are brand new
Some are very old
Some are tranquil
Some are bold
Some are favorites
Some are cast-outs
Some mix well
Some don't

But the box is the common bond
That holds everyone together, and
When the crayons are used together,
They can create beauty and love.

Realizing that these last chapters were a bit on the serious side, I would like to leave you with one more story. I hope it puts a smile on your face.

Time-Out

As you have now come to know through the bulk of these stories, our little Greer is a handful. She does the unexpected almost daily. She makes us laugh, cry and wring our hands in frustration. She could test the patience of a saint.

Greer looks like a pixie with twinkling eyes, an infectious smile and freckles—which she calls sprinkles—across her nose. She is tiny but has a fearless, take-no-prisoners attitude.

I believe the fight to survive after her premature birth has given her strength beyond her years, and she will become something amazing when she matures.

I can't wait.

When Greer was going through her terrible twos, I wasn't sure who was going to survive, Greer or her parents. Most of the time my money was on Greer.

Because of her unyielding behavior, terrible tantrums and lack of reasoning at her young age, disciplining her was a huge problem. The only solution that seemed to work—and allowed her to vent her frustration and eventually calm down—was to place her in her high chair.

There Greer could be secured and the tray across her lap would bear the brunt of her outbursts. This chair was the only place where she could be confined for a brief period of time-out when she had done something that wasn't allowed.

One particular day, she had done something to one of her sisters. Greer was told she had to go to time-out and she was not liking it one bit.

It took both parents to get her into the high chair to let her vent. And vent she did.

If my son-in-law Bradley had not recorded this with his smart phone, I would not have believed the tantrum from this tiny little thing.

Starting off, Greer was red-faced and crying. Her short hair was all messed up and she was banging on the tray of her high chair and screaming at her daddy.

The conversation at this point was somewhat one-sided. Greer was doing all the talking and making most of the demands.

I could hear some chuckling in the background. I mean what else can you do with this? I could only hear Greer's side of the conversation but what I remember, the end of the tantrum went something like this.

"I don't want to go to time-out! No! *You* go live with Nana! This is *my* house! *Capiche*!"

Now, I don't know about you, but it sounded to me like going to Nana's house was a bad thing. I can't imagine that was one of her punishment options. My only conclusion to that comment was that Greer had pretty much broken her parents at that point. They were seriously considering shipping her off to me.

Imagine that.

As much as their parents may think otherwise, I will have you know that Greer, as well as the other grandchildren, think coming to Nana's house is pretty awesome.

And they should.

No matter how big or how old The Grands get, I will be there for each of them with a twinkle in my eyes, open arms and a smile on my face.

Always.

Grandchildren give us a second chance to do things better because they bring out the best in us.

— Author Unknown

Acknowledgements

I wish to thank my sweet daughters and their husbands, Kristy and Brant, and Jenny and Bradley, who so graciously allowed me to share with the world true stories about their families. Their children were my inspiration, and I could not have written this book without them.

Also, much gratitude to Kristy, Jenny, Renee, Linda and Rhonda for their contributions to the review and edit process. Many thanks also to family and friends who contributed grandparent titles.

And to Elizabeth Fisher, who was my rock from beginning to end. Her layout expertise was invaluable.

Artist Lisa Haggerty Palmer provided me with another incredible cover. Her talent is amazing and her heart is pure gold.

Also, I wish to thank up-and-coming young artist (and granddaughter), Allie R., for her colorful interpretation of Nana. I am very proud of you.

Finally, I want to thank my husband, Russell, for his patience, encouragement and love during this incredible, late-in-life adventure of mine. He has never allowed me to give up, even when discouragement seemed to be lurking around every corner. Thanks for always being there for me. I love you. JG

Made in the USA
Charleston, SC
13 November 2014